Soaring Above Adversity

"Mr. Bugg took wonderful care of his wife during a difficult and prolonged illness. This book is the inspirational story of a family's journey and can provide guidance to others that are facing a similar path."

Priscilla Callahan-Lyon, MD

"An insightful personal testimony. Takes you along on this care giver's journey through both the heart-warming moments and tearful challenges that are part of taking care of someone living with Alzheimer's disease. This book serves as a valuable resource for families dealing with the daily demands of this long-term—and still incurable—illness."
RaeAnn E. Butler, MBA, NHA

Administrator
Edenton Retirement Community

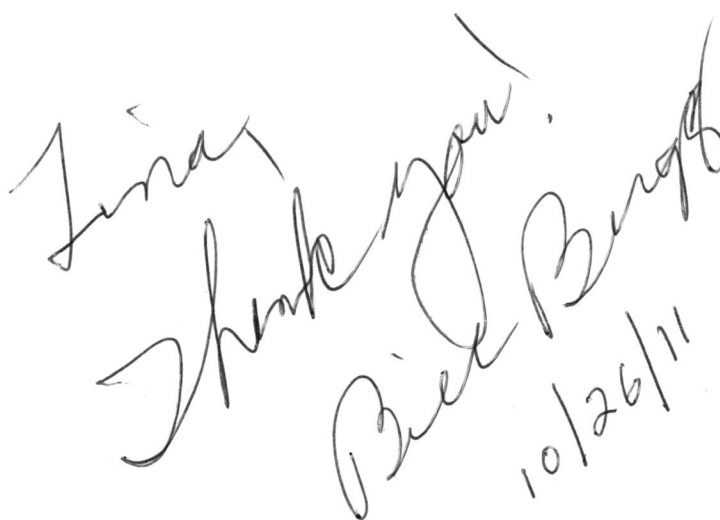

Soaring Above Adversity

By

Bill Bugg

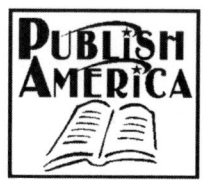

PublishAmerica
Baltimore

© 2007 by Bill Bugg.
All rights reserved. No part of this book may be reproduced, stored in a retrieval system or transmitted in any form or by any means without the prior written permission of the publishers, except by a reviewer who may quote brief passages in a review to be printed in a newspaper, magazine or journal.

First printing

At the specific preference of the author, PublishAmerica allowed this work to remain exactly as the author intended, verbatim, without editorial input.

ISBN: 1-4241-0880-2
PUBLISHED BY PUBLISHAMERICA, LLLP
www.publishamerica.com
Baltimore

Printed in the United States of America

This book is dedicated to the memory

Of my wife Billie Jean whose long battle

With Alzheimer's inspired me to write

The book for the benefit of others.

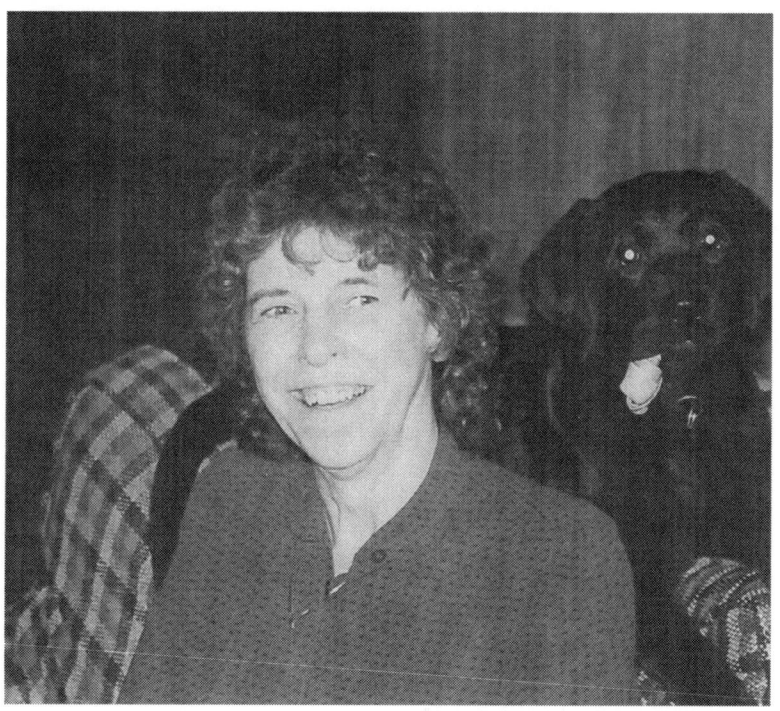

Billie Jean and Bear

Contents

Introduction 7

Chapter 1: Alzheimer's, the Beginning to the End 9
Chapter 2: Spiritual Recognition 34
    "Footprints in the Sand" by Mary Stevenson 45
Chapter 3: The Power of Positive Thinking 46
Chapter 4: Legal and Administrative Needs 67
Chapter 5: Building and Protecting Your Assets 83
Chapter 6: Staying Mentally and Physically Fit 100
Conclusion 119

Appendix A 122

Introduction

I painfully watched my wife waste away over eighteen years with Alzheimer's. I did all I could to help her, to care for her and to keep her as happy as possible. Throughout those eighteen years I was still able to cope and to enjoy many of the good things life has to offer. I am writing this book based on what I learned as the caregiver for my wife during those eighteen years and based on some of my experiences that allowed me to cope as the caregiver to my wife. My intent for the book is to be helpful and informative in relating some of those experiences and in relating the things I learned that are needed in caring for a loved one with Alzheimer's or any other disease or occurrence that cripples the person beyond being self reliant.

I will discuss my experiences from the initial recognition of her disease symptoms to her passing. I found that spiritual recognition as well as a reliance on positive thinking helped me get through many tough times. Alzheimer's in a family member presents many struggles and a realization that a longer life together intended in earlier years will not become a reality. The devastation to plans made long ago occurs with many other diseases in loved ones. It is then very necessary for everyone to accomplish the needs required to ease the threat of adversity and the occurrence of adversity before any adversity occurs. The needs I will address are obtaining and keeping updated necessary documents like wills, trusts and powers-of-attorney; obtaining the insurance types you will need; investing to help insure finances will be available to care for a handicapped loved one; keeping mentally and physically fit.

I hope you will find the book meets my intent of being helpful and informative and a benefit whether you are now experiencing some adversity in your life or not. The book will be useful to young as well as older readers through coverage of some things best accomplished in the younger years. My ordeal was much more manageable because I had accomplished the legal and financial needs before my wife was stricken with Alzheimer's.

The book has been reviewed for technical accuracy by a medical doctor, an attorney, a certified financial planner, an assisted living facility administrator and a minister.

It will help to have pencil and paper ready to make notes as you read this book. I list more books in the appendix which I found to be very helpful to me even before my wife was diagnosed with Alzheimer's.

Chapter 1
Alzheimer's, the Beginning to the End

Let's start at the beginning, when you first start noticing some little, subtle change in a friend or family member. I say a friend because it is very possible that a friend will notice some change in a person before a family member. Bringing that up with a family member could help bring faster diagnosis and treatment if Alzheimer's is present in the beginning stages. That is important because there are medications that may help slow the progression of Alzheimer's in some patients. For patients whom the drugs work, the earlier they start taking these drugs the longer the disease may be slowed.

My wife started with some very minor lapses in memory, little things like not remembering some points in a conversation after it had just taken place. We family members, not even thinking about Alzheimer's had our own reactions to her minor memory lapses. I would get irritated and tell her she needed to pay more attention particularly if I thought she had forgotten something important. Our daughter would respond to some instances of forgetfulness by saying things like, "Mom, we just talked about that," not in an arrogant way but showing frustration at why her mother was becoming so forgetful.

Even though her ability to remember things got worse, the progress in my wife was slow enough that none of us thought of Alzheimer's, we remained aloof to her situation believing, or at least hoping, the problem would go away. These memory lapses also started when my wife was only fifty years old. This is another reason we didn't consider Alzheimer's as the cause.

A very close friend and neighbor cornered me one day and said my wife had come to see her worried about her problem remembering things. I now felt very bad at not paying more attention to my wife's problem. I now realized she was concerned and had confided in someone else probably because of the way I had not taken her memory loss seriously. I mention this so you will not duplicate my very incorrect way of handling the initial memory loss of a family member or friend. I believe in the every day rush of events my initial reaction may be typical for others so again, please do pay attention to minor but recurring forgetting or any other on-going change taking place in your loved ones. Having been given the "heads up" I did begin to pay more attention and surely became sympathetic instead of antagonistic toward my wife's problem.

So you can see I learned the hard way one rule of thumb for determining Alzheimer's and that is to not ignore even the most minor forgetfulness if it is repetitive. Another rule of thumb is to notice what is being forgotten. At times we all forget where we put the car keys but forgetting what the car keys are used for or even what they are is a sign of a much more significant problem.

Another sign prevalent in the beginning of Alzheimer's is

the person will ask the same question multiple times in the span of a few short minutes each time having forgotten the answer they were given.

Please though do not become upset and make your own errant diagnosis of Alzheimer's over small incidents of forgetfulness. Just make a mental note and monitor the situation. Remember, while the incidence of Alzheimer's is increasing, it occurs in less than ten percent of the population today, and there are other curable causes of memory loss. The ten percent is for the entire population regardless of age. As we age, the percent of the population with Alzheimer's increases.

Also do not make disparaging or angry remarks to the person who can't remember. It is better initially to just try to ease the concern of the person who is forgetful. Just be sure to make note of the occurrence and see if it repeats itself on an ongoing and increasing basis.

My wife's forgetting became increasingly repetitive. Initially she did not forget things like cooking a meal or driving a car but she was forgetting things like what just happened on a TV program or some things she had done that day. This supports the fact that early memory loss with Alzheimer's is of short term occurrences. Longer term memory loss comes later in the progression of the disease.

Another early sign of Alzheimer's is the beginning of changes in personality. My wife began to show some minor but noticeable changes in her personality. She was a relatively introverted person who was becoming more extroverted. One change she was demonstrating was faster to get angry, anger at not being able to remember or to do the things she had done for years, eventually some since being a child. She also became more outspoken over little things, things she normally ignored. So now the two things, short term memory loss and personality changes, which are the definite signals that Alzheimer's is present were occurring in my wife.

My wife was working as a secretary during these early stages of memory loss. I wondered if what I was noticing at home was also being noticed at her office. On checking with a friend who worked with her I found out it was. In fact the company she worked for eventually had to downsize and my wife was terminated from her job. I was angry at that since I believed and still believe she should have been offered disability. I, though, needed to have been more involved in what she was doing at work so I could have perhaps prompted a release due to disability instead of out right severance. So if your spouse or some other loved one is working when the memory loss starts please make a call to the person's boss or the company's personnel department if they have one so maybe you can get a better resolution then my wife got.

As the signs of forgetting and personality changes progressed I decided it was time to have her physician determine the cause of her forgetfulness. The first testing he did was to ask her a series of questions and note the answers. These tests are called mini-mental exams. On the next visit he asked the same questions and noted the answers. There was a grade associated with the answers given and after a period of several months when those grades continued to decrease her physician sent her for numerous other tests to determine the cause of her memory loss. These initially involved blood tests, x-rays and other tests all toward ruling out any other problem like chemical imbalances or other medical illness that could be producing the symptoms other than Alzheimer's. As these tests results all came back negative there was one final test administered. This test was by a psychologist. The test amounted to having my wife answer some questions, remember certain word sequences and copy some drawings like a square or a circle. My wife knew none of the answers to the questions. Questions like what is the day of the week, the year. She remembered none of the word sequences like remembering three words that could be colors. In less than a minute she could remember none of the words. In trying to draw a circle she became so agitated she threw the pencil across the room because she had no idea where to begin even though the picture of a circle was right in front of her. The result of this final test and the results of all the previous testing left no answer except she had Alzheimer's.

The results of this final test was also an awakening to me that my wife was really sick. When she had no idea how to start to draw a circle that was right in front of her was a real shock to me. More than anything before that I now knew I had an extremely difficult situation to handle with no idea what to do or where to start. There was then also a realization that I now was going to be effectively without my best friend, lover and companion for the rest of my life.

At that point I contacted the local Alzheimer's Association for help. The Alzheimer's Association is in many towns and cities across the United States. Getting in touch with them is as easy as looking for their phone number in the phone book. They sent me several books, more on me caring for me as the main caregiver than on what needed to be done for my wife. For her safety, there were instructions on how to accident proof the home all of which I installed. Things like putting an out-of sight on/off switch on the electric stove; barricading inside stairs, putting non-skid liners on the inside and outside steps; using night lights in bathrooms and halls; install grab bars and any other safety measure in bathrooms to prevent the person from falling; and storing all sharp objects out of sight. I later learned that I also had to put a latch on the outside of the gate that leads from our yard. Twice my wife walked out and was roaming down the street when fortunately, both times, a neighbor saw her and brought her home. Keeping your loved one safe at home is a priority that must be constantly exercised.

Another thing the Alzheimer's Association made me aware of was their support for enrolling Alzheimer's patients in the Safe Return program. This program allows you to register information about your loved one so if they are ever lost by wandering away others like law enforcement agencies can identify the person and contact the responsible person to get them and bring them home. I enrolled my wife in this program without hesitation.

One of many mistakes I made in caring for my wife was in letting her drive too long. I had several people tell me that taking away independence from a loved one as Alzheimer's progresses is one of the most difficult things to do. I was finding that to be true so my intent was to give her all the independence I could to lessen the impact she would experience as she lost her independence over time. Her driving also lessened the impact on me as there was some driving she did that I did not have to do. Even though I now knew she had Alzheimer's I had not adjusted to the real consequences to me, the person who had to become her main caregiver. This, I suppose, is a form of denial, not at the fact my wife had the disease but what it was really going to require from me.

Allowing her to still drive was a bad decision in any case. I was home one day and received a phone call from a realtor at a new housing development. My wife had gone to a place she had visited for several years but made a wrong turn on the way home and ended up scared and twenty miles from home. At least she still had the ability to stop and tell someone she was lost. I went to get her and she was able to follow me home and shortly after had no recollection of the incident. This happened one more time when she was returning home from the same place. She made a wrong turn and this time someone called me from a phone booth thirty miles away saying my wife was there and lost. Again I went to get her but after this time I made the very difficult decision she had to stop driving. This decision was for her safety but I felt terrible at taking away yet another part of her independence. She never once complained about not driving. I believe she may have remotely remembered being afraid when she got lost but mostly I believe she did not complain because she had forgotten those incidents and did not remember what driving was.

For me as the main caregiver, I was constantly faced with the determination of when to eliminate things from my wife's life for her protection. This coupled with the every day awareness that someone you love and has been with you for many years, we were married for forty seven years at the time of her death, is slowly leaving you is difficult to take. I continually had to realize I still had my life and while my wife was my number one responsibility I did have to keep going and doing enjoyable things. This also allowed me to be at my best in caring for my wife. In subsequent chapters of this book I will cover some of the things that helped me get through the ordeal I was having to handle on a daily basis.

Being at your best is a point of great significance for all the members of the family but particularly for the main caregiver. As the main caregiver you are in a situation that wasn't your choice, not familiar to you, for which most of us have no training and which is beginning to occupy more and more of your time. Of course, the toughest realization is your loved one is slowly leaving you and there is nothing you can do except make them as comfortable and well cared for as possible. Then you must face the reality there is nothing you can do to stop the disease and make plans to insure your life is not put at risk through sorrow, depression, worry, guilt or anything else. These harmful emotions will greatly reduce your capability to care for your loved one in the best possible way. All of your decisions will be less than adequate when these negative emotions are occupying much of your thinking.

Be sure you make time for things you the caregiver need and enjoy to maintain your physical and mental health. More and more of your time will have to be spent at home as the disease worsens in your loved one. I started several things to keep me occupied at home. One was to make and plant multiple gardens around the yard. I gave each a theme and installed statuary and lighting. This activity gave me something to do, kept me occupied and kept me busy at home where I could care for my wife. In addition, I began to remove the "get around to its" that had been lingering over time, some for years. These things for me are enjoyable. In the same circumstances you would need to pick things that are enjoyable to you and get started doing them.

Now, returning to my wife's care, I had a job that required me to be away from home for almost a week every other week. I would prepare my wife's dinners on individual plates before

I left. This way I could include the things she liked to eat, as opposed to store bought prepared dinners. She could still get my prepared dinners from the refrigerator and put them in the microwave. Eventually, I had to get a microwave that had a one-button control marked for prepared dinners. I put a bright colored piece of tape on that control and for a while longer she could still heat her home made dinners by pressing one button.

Using the phone also became a chore for her so I initially posted the important numbers beside the phone but later I had to get a phone that allowed one-button dialing by storing the important numbers. I put a piece of tape with the names of those persons on the button for their preset number. This all worked until the phone company decided we had to dial the area code before the number for local calls. Phones at that time did not allow storing all those numbers and those that did required a one first to designate long distance. Use of the phone became another of her lost privileges adding to my wife's loss of independence.

As my wife's disease continued to worsen I found I needed some in-home care for my wife when I was away at work. I was becoming more concerned about her being alone in the house where she was increasingly unable to do much for herself. My children were helping as much as possible but they and their spouses worked and they also had their families to care for. I got a list of in-home care organizations from the Alzheimer's Association and did some amount of investigation to try to pick good ones. I'd have to say my experience was not very good with either of the organizations I selected. The first one sent young people who really took no time to care for my wife. They would show up, sit in another room away from my wife and told me they were not to touch the patient. That turned out to be an eleven dollar per hour study hall and baby sitting service. I then went to a hospital that supplied people for in-home care to sign up for their service figuring that someone who was associated with a hospital would at least be able to do something for the patient. Wrong! And this time it was costing me eleven dollars and fifty cents an hour. I decided this approach to getting the help my wife needed was not going to work.

Soon after this, by making phone calls and talking to others, networking in other words, I learned there are day care centers that will care for physically and mentally challenged adults. I found a great one. Not only were they caring and good, they picked my wife up at home each morning and brought her back each afternoon. When I was not traveling on business this also allowed me time to get away from home chores, like grocery shopping, done as well as have some respite.

We continued like this until I returned home from one of my business trips to find each of the four dinners I had prepared still in the refrigerator. Thank goodness I would also leave buns and candy on the counter that my wife liked as snacks because that is all she had eaten for four days. It now became obvious that I could not leave her alone while I was away. My bad experiences with in-home care organizations left me groping for answers. Either I had to leave my job or find someone who could care for my wife all day while I was away.

I'd found previously in locating the day care center that networking works. Now, for the second time, I needed to network to find an in-home professional care taker several days a week. These caretakers are very different from my previous experiences as they are usually nurses or people with similar skills who often work independent of any organization. They are also usually more expensive.

I began asking everyone I knew and most I met whether they knew anyone that did in-home care for Alzheimer's patients. I had become friends with the driver and owner of the airport transportation service I used to get to and from the airports for my business trips. I mentioned my dilemma to him one day and he said his Mother had cared in home for a gentleman who had Alzheimer's. He thought she would like to do that again. She would and did. This lady was nothing short of a miracle for me and for my wife. She came each day I was away and fed my wife, took her to the malls and to see the horse she, the caretaker, owned. They became real buddies. My wife called her "my girl". I still fixed the dinners and put them in the refrigerator but I had no more worries that she would not be eating them. In addition, I could feel good that someone who knew much more than I knew about caring for an Alzheimer's patient was in charge while I was away. My wife could still be trusted to stay in bed and to sleep until her caregiver arrived each morning.

This arrangement continued for a year or so until it began to become obvious that my wife could no longer stay alone at nights. Our care giver said she would be glad to stay all day and night every day while I was away but I felt not only was that an imposition on her, she had a family at home, it would become a great expense for me. Several years before this I had purchased long term care insurance for my wife and me. I mistakenly did not take in-home care as a part of the policy so having a person spend full time with my wife at home was going to get very expensive.

Given this new dilemma I sat down and closely evaluated my financial situation. After doing that and having several conversations with my family and financial advisor I decided I could resign from my job. I was making good money but the rising cost of caring for my wife and my desire to be home with her more, made that decision relatively easy.

Maybe your initial financial evaluation of your assets won't allow you to resign from your job but make sure you are thorough in your evaluation. You may find you can retire and take a part time job to supplement your retirement income which can include social security, any pension you may receive and contributions from your savings. If you have in-home care coverage in your long term care policy that will help provide the financial coverage you need to be away from home in a job while your loved one is cared for by an in-home professional. That will also allow you time for some respite.

In addition, in your financial evaluation do not forget your spouse may be eligible to soon receive Social Security or will continue to receive Social Security if he or she is currently receiving it.

Do not forget to include an evaluation of your loved one's assets to qualify for Medicaid if you find a lack of finances will not allow you to retire. With Medicaid, if your loved one qualifies, your loved one will be able to enter an outside the home care facility where they will be cared for while you continue to be employed. If your loved one can qualify for Medicaid be sure to get on the waiting list at several facilities and on the waiting list for receiving Medicaid.

Having your time freed to be home as much as possible to care for your loved one will be a great benefit to you and to your loved one.

My wife had progressed past the point of being cared for in a day-care facility which are not usually staffed to handle things like incontinence and the inability of attendees to feed themselves. This meant I now had to dress her and put her to bed. I did the cooking, fed her and changed her diaper. I did everything any parent has to do for a young infant twenty four hours a day, seven days a week. I did hire a person to come once a week to clean the house. That gave me a few hours to go out for groceries and other needed items. That was also some brief respite for me.

I want to make a couple of points here. One is the type of diapers to use. First I bought the kind that stick together on the sides. This type could separate and the sticky part would stick to my wife's skin causing much irritation. I looked for the slip on kind, the ones that go on like panties. I could not find them at the time so I continually had to check that there was no irritation.

Another point is how often to check to see if a diaper was soiled. If I waited too long there would be an irritation from that and, at times, a mess in the chair so I had to perform a diaper check every two hours.

I was becoming very dissatisfied with my ability to care for my wife in the best way. I was learning "on the job" but knew I was not learning a lot of what was needed to give my wife the best possible life for her condition. That surely was not the best thing for my wife so I started asking everyone who I thought would know something about Alzheimer's patients if they thought she was ready for an assisting living facility or nursing home. I talked to her doctor, the Alzheimer's Association, nursing homes, my family and her past care providers. All, without exception, agreed she needed to be in a home. The best reason came from the supervisor at the day care center my wife had attended. She told me that my wife still had some ability to form a relationship but that would probably not last much longer. She said if my wife went to a facility after losing that ability it would be much harder for her to adapt to the changed environment.

Other considerations in making the decision for in-facility care are the safety of your home and does the person fall down often, my wife fell twice, both times being injured; how good are you in maintaining good personal hygiene for the patient; is the person's behavior becoming more than you can handle; are you sure the person is getting enough of the proper foods and liquids; are you able to amuse the person with things they can still perform. Given all of this and occurrences like her falling twice and hurting herself I now went shopping for a nursing home or long term care facility. This was another task for which I had no previous training or experience.

I looked at nursing homes and assisted living facilities, what each provided in the way of care and the varying costs each required. I found, as suggested by the Alzheimer's Association literature I had requested, that walking unannounced into a facility works well. I suggest you go around lunch time and ask to see someone from admissions. Be sure to get a guided tour around the entire part of the facility where your loved one would be housed and cared for. Observe the patients rooms, private or shared, and the conditions in those rooms. Are they clean and safe? For example, is there a sprinkler system, a firewall barrier, a fire alarm system and smoke detectors. Your overall evaluation of facilities needs to include the environment, staff ratios, frequency and type of activities, who conducts the activities, meals and specialty programs particularly geared to the varying patient limitations as the patient's memory loss grows worse.

The type of room to select is also a consideration. Based on my experience, I recommend a shared room. First, the patient is probably not going to notice or care whether the room has someone else in there or not. This is particularly true if the patient is being admitted at the point they require out-of-home professional help. Second, until they are completely bed ridden they will probably spend very little time in the room unless sleeping and third, the shared rooms are usually substantially less expensive than private rooms. There are some facilities though that only have private rooms. The assisted living facility I eventually selected only had private rooms but the cost was in line with other facilities shared rooms.

I realize the tendency for family members will be to select a private room because that is what they would select for themselves. The family members, though, need to be aware of the condition of their loved one and make prudent decisions for them. This is particularly true for those families who may be struggling with the decision to commit their loved one because of the financial burden imposed by the costs.

On your tour of each facility you visit, observe the rest rooms and the bathing area. Check the kitchen and dining area and if you are there during the serving of a meal note the food being served and particularly note the assistance the patients needing feeding assistance are receiving. Insure the Alzheimer's unit has secured doors to prevent the patients from voluntarily leaving the area. Ask about the procedure for giving medications, what is the medical emergency procedure, what is the evacuation procedure in case of fire or other emergencies.

Get all the printed information the facility has to offer for later reading. You will need this to help you compare facilities as well as to develop other questions you will want to have answered later. Go over costs in detail, understand what is included or not included in each cost item. For example, I had to purchase diapers, surgical gloves and baby wipes. These were not covered in any of the other facility costs. The facility would have gotten these things for me but I would be billed. I found I could get the items cheaper in bulk elsewhere.

After determining the total cost at several facilities you may need to use that information to do another complete financial analysis of your situation as you may have done to determine if you could retire. As I said before when considering retirement, if finances are going to be a problem now again examine all possibilities that will allow your loved one to be admitted to a facility. You may need to see an attorney in this case to help you evaluate whether your loved one is Medicaid eligible or what needs to be done for them to become Medicaid eligible. If Medicaid will be used be sure to check which of the facilities will accept it. Most nursing homes will accept Medicaid while assisted living facilities will not but Medicaid varies from state to state and the type of facilities accepting it may also vary. You can get more information from your state or county office on aging.
Notice I am talking about Medicaid and not Medicare. Medicare will not cover any costs associated with long term care needs beyond a few days.
Having enough long term care insurance will ease the financial worry and allow most people to virtually disregard the subject of finances as a problem in determining to admit their loved one to in-facility care. Long term care insurance will be covered more thoroughly in chapter five.

Differences in nursing homes and assisted living facilities also need to be examined and understood especially if finances are a problem since nursing homes are generally much more expensive. The differences in nursing homes and assisted living facilities are primarily determined by the state licensing requirements which in turn determine the type and extent of services and care provided. A phone call to the state health department will get you to a person who can tell you what the licensing differences are in your state. In my state I found that typically assisted living facilities are rated at three levels, level one, two or three. Level three facilities are usually very close to nursing homes and will provide the needed care for an Alzheimer's patient until they pass on, usually at less cost. The assisted living facility I chose did.

When you have narrowed your selection of a long term care facility to a few, before making the final choice, you need to call each potential selection and schedule at least one half day at the facility with your loved one. Be sure that the time there includes a meal so you can observe your loved one's reactions and the support from the staff. Have the activities director who will be directing your loved ones activities meet with you and discuss some of these activities. Being able to observe these activities in progress is even better. Also talk to the on duty nurse about the procedures in place for notifying you if your loved one seems to be experiencing pain or if they become physically ill.

You will need to add your name to the waiting list of each facility you visit. You can have your name removed from the waiting list of facilities you do not pick at the time you make that decision.

After going through all of these evaluations it is time to select the facility you want your loved one to move in to. Having already been on the facility waiting list it should only be a matter of a short time before you will be moving your loved one in. There will be a contract to sign so get a copy of it so you can read it thoroughly and develop questions you want answered before signing it. Get the answers to all of your questions before the move in time arrives. Soon you will get a call that there is a room available and you need to sign the contract. There are a few other items to now tend to.

Most facilities have their own physician on call. I decided to stay with my wife's physician since she had all the records and first-hand knowledge of my wife's medical history. I made sure the assisted living facility I selected would keep a record of all the contact information needed to get immediate first hand answers to questions they had about my wife's physical health. Of course my wife's physician was also aware of the need to be responsive to these requests and she was excellent and timely in her responses. The use of fax machines was very beneficial.

In further support of this arrangement of keeping my wife's physician I had to drive my wife about thirty miles to see her physician every three months but that was good. It gave her a chance to get out of the facility and it gave me direct input on my wife's condition as her disease progressed. In fact this arrangement worked so well I highly recommend you stay with your loved one's physician instead of having the facility use their on-call physician. In this case you need to insure the facility gets your permission before calling in any other physician unless it is an emergency. I usually okayed requests for visits to trim finger and toe nails or to do x-rays when my wife had done something to raise suspicion she may have an injury.

Prior to entering the facility I was concerned my wife was getting to the point of not being able to tell of any pain she may be experiencing so before having her enter a facility I took her for a complete physical. I took her to the dentist to make sure her teeth were not at the point of causing pain. I took her to the ophthalmologist to ensure her eyes were fine as they were currently corrected.

The visit to check her eyes really was not effective since her disease had progressed to the point of her not being able to remember long enough to tell the doctor which of the lens was better. If you want to have your loved one checked for their vision I suggest you do that early in the stages of the disease. Actually, not long after being in the facility my wife lost her glasses but it really had no effect on her daily happiness. She had gotten to the point of not reading or paying attention to television so the loss of her glasses turned out to be not important.

There is also something I learned from the trip to the dentist. The dental assistant was holding a piece of gauze in my wife's mouth and told her to close. She did, very tightly, catching one of the assistant's fingers inside. When the assistant told her to open my wife only bore down harder since she could no longer determine open from close. When the dentist finally got my wife's mouth open there was enough damage to the assistant's finger that she needed to put ice on it. Therefore, when you take your loved one to the dentist please alert the dentist and the assistant that they need to be aware that open and close may not have a recognizable difference to the patient.

Preparing to move your loved one to a facility is very heart breaking for the entire family. The move-in day is a day filled with emotion and tears. When the time came to move my wife I did have the support of my family. My son and son-in-law helped me with the move.

I could have had the room totally furnished with the facilities furniture but as you can imagine it resembled the furniture of a hospital room without the personal touches. I decided to move some of our furniture in as well as several of the items I thought my wife could identify with including pictures. While the room looked good I believe it was more for my family and me because I do not believe what was in the room made any difference to my wife. The disease had progressed to that extent. Also, she spent no time during her waking hours in the room.

Another consideration as to what is in the room concerns the behavior of other residents. There are some who when gaining access to the room will break items, sometimes by just dropping them, things like pictures. At other times some of the residents will purposefully break items by throwing them or will take them for their own. Getting a taken item away from some residents is not an easy task so be cautious about what you put in the room whether the room is private or shared.

My wife did acclimate to the facility over not too much time. This was enhanced by the attention she was being given particularly by the social director in her unit at the time of her admission. My wife did continue to form relationships with the entire facility staff which true to the advice I had received helped immensely in her feeling accepted. She seemed to take to most of the staff and they to her which really helped her keep her smile. She called the staff members "my people". Her expression of dissatisfaction to me on what was happening to her on the day of the move was quickly replaced by smiles on most of my subsequent visits. This was a big relief for me.

My family and I would take her out to dinner and after a while I would bring her home for visits. I waited several weeks before bringing her home because I was afraid of causing her undue grief if she were to visit her home too soon after entering the facility and remembered it was her home. Our efforts were to use the word "home" to refer to her new surroundings, indeed her new home. This turned out to be a really good idea and she did get to the point where home for her was in the facility. In fact after some amount of time we had to stop taking her out to go anywhere other than to see her doctor because she would get very nervous being in strange surroundings including her previous home.

I visited her several times a week and I recommend you do the same for your loved one for several reasons. One is to ensure the staff is caring for your loved one in the manner you require. You are paying a lot of money for your loved one's care and you need to make sure the best possible care is being provided. You also need to insure un-needed care is not being provided at an extra charge. There was one time the facility medical staff thought it would be good for my wife to see a psychiatrist. I didn't understand this since she could not comprehend questions much less answer them. The psychiatrist's assistant was there when I next visited and had seen my wife. Given her recommendations I merely answered her recommendations for "treatment" with a response it would be fine but I would not pay for any of it. None of the recommendations were performed and my wife was no worse off. I relate this to impress on the care giver and all family members that being active in your loved ones new environment and involved with their everyday activities is very necessary for your loved one and the entire family to insure the proper care is being administered on a regular basis and to insure unneeded extra cost care is not being provided.

Another reason to visit frequently is at times there may be staff members who are not doing the job they are supposed to do. I had instances where this was the case. I would immediately inform the administrator of the facility who always resolved the problem quickly. Do not hesitate to express your concerns and bring up problems. They cannot be solved if they are not known to the personnel at the facility who can solve them.

I went so far at one point to look into another facility because I believed the care for my wife had deteriorated. Before making any change I had a meeting with the administrator and other key people responsible for my wife's care. That meeting resolved the problems. You would need to do the same thing before moving your loved one. As I have said my wife had become very acclimated to her surroundings and I believe any permanent move could have been very upsetting to her. With the infrequent lapses in care she was receiving I believe the facility I chose was a good facility and did a good job in caring for her. I would select that same facility today.

The very positive responsiveness I received from the facility administrator when I became concerned about my wife's care was a big help to me so, to repeat, I recommend that you do not hesitate to go to the top person whenever you believe your loved one is getting less than the best care.

The more important reason for frequent visits is to see your loved one. Even if some visits can only be for a few minutes you have helped brighten the day for your loved one and some of the other residents. On many visits I brought our Labrador Retriever to see her and some of the other residents. I noticed that several residents at the facility seemed to never have a visitor.

Let me repeat here that while the main purpose of your visit is to see your loved one and have them see you, do not neglect the other residents. I found most of them loved some attention and loved my dog. Most important for me was the real satisfaction I got from visiting with my wife and her new family of friends. It's amazing the therapy I got from helping someone else smile. I think my dog also got some of that same therapy because his tail never stopped wagging while he was there. There were many experiences that brought not just smiles to my and the staff's face but outright laughter.

For example, one ninety two year old preacher's wife who was confined to a wheelchair, I'll call her Mary, could be nice one day and very cantankerous the next day but her cutting wit was ever present. On one of her cantankerous days I was attempting to get her to smile but each attempt brought a deeper scowl. Finally, having enough of me, she said, "You're a wimp. My husband would make ten of you." I said, "I know Mary but I was hoping you could help me get better." She replied, "Go to hell, you're not worth it." Even the laughter from the rest of us did not remove her scowl.

Then there was Jean, a retired nurse and patient who was initially assigned to my wife to help her acclimate to her new surroundings. One day at lunch my wife was particularly upset and Jean reached over, patted her arm and said, "That's all right honey, at least you have someone here with you. My two sons brought me here, opened the door and threw me in and now they're in my house taking women into my bed." Needless to say that not only brought loud laughter but also helped me hide my tears at my wife's earlier tears.

Alice had been on a farm all her life. She had cows she had to call from the meadow and feed. Alice could be very aggressive but one thing that would settle her down was to tell her the cows needed to be called into the barn. Alice would then loudly call, "whooooop cows, whooooop cows," until she was told all the cows were in. She called so loud I was sure that if any cows were within a mile of the facility they'd be in the barn now.

While these folks memories continue to fade and recognition of others seems to disappear I always wondered what may be going on back somewhere in their brains that they just could not get to come out. I strongly suggest you and the entire family visit your loved one and the others often and not just for one or two annual occasions. You'll actually be the one who, I believe, receives the most benefit in the long run. I surely did and I know my dog also must have some good memories of the visits as well.

There are some who say it's difficult to see a spouse, parent, child or close friend in whatever the person's condition has become. My answer is, "Yes, it is most difficult." but not going to see the person is much worse. Here is a family member or friend who may well have some recognition that some family member, relative or friend is not coming to see them and I cringe to imagine the hurt that may well be imbedded in the patient with no ability to express that hurt.

There were times I left following a visit with my wife with tears hardly able to stay in my eyes until I could get out of the door. My drive home was through blurred vision. Most often though, my visits were very uplifting for me because I was able to bring some little smile or other reaction that I knew had brought some happy thought from somewhere back in the recesses of my wife's brain. Many times these favorable reactions were brought on by distractions like bringing my dog, doing a little skit, dancing a jig or looking at pictures. Even though at times my wife did not seem to know me she still seemed to recognize some delight or humor from some activity.

Several times during her several years in the home our band would play for an event like the Christmas party. The first few times the band was there my wife would get up and start dancing to the delight of everyone.

I would hope if you have any thoughts of not going to see your loved one frequently you strongly "suck it up" and go make those visits. It is a fact that Alzheimer's patients will eventually get to the point of not recognizing anyone, all family members included. This fact nor most anything else is a viable excuse not to go to visit. Surely your loved one has been through much difficulty and is experiencing even more difficulty coping with their problem than you will experience visiting. After all you get to leave and go on with your life. Your loved one has lost that choice.

Chapter 2
Spiritual Recognition

We all have our trials and tribulations, our adversities and most of us have our God, whatever our religion, who is a part of our lives to help us get through those trying times in our lives. Often though we do not recognize that God does prepare us for things that will occur in our future. I am thankful that I have been able to realize that recognition of God's work in my life. There were four events in my life that I initially did not see as the primary preparation I would receive to help me get through the most horrendous event of my life, my wife's eighteen year bout with Alzheimer's.

The first event started twenty five years ago when my physician at the time approached me and asked if I would like to join him in an organization that was based on multi-level marketing. I did join with the original purpose to make money by selling products and to train others to also sell those same products. The people I became associated with in that organization were very much oriented toward positive thinking and the partaking of books and tapes that endorsed, encouraged and taught ways to become a positive thinker.

God was also at the center of their happiness and He is at the center of making positive thinking available to all whom will take the time to understand the benefits of being positive. More on the benefits of positive thinking will be covered in chapter three.

At the start of my association with this group of people I had lost my eagerness to read much of anything having spent many years in school. I first studied veterinary medicine and then transferred to engineering. I completed all the class work for a doctorate in engineering and I had completed all the reading that required. I welcomed the opportunity not to have to read any more books except as needed to accomplish my job. But in the organization I joined I couldn't help but notice how happy the people were. They were always smiling and seemed to be able to handle the obstacles that came their way.

When I asked how most of these people could always seem to be so happy and in control I was told that if I would begin to read some of their suggested positive thinking materials for just fifteen minutes a night it would prove very beneficial to me. I decided that fifteen minutes is not a very long time so I purchased one of their recommended books. After a few nights of reading for fifteen minutes I found I was reading twenty minutes, then thirty minutes, then one hour. I purchased more of the books and read more, purchased more books and read more. Soon people began to say to me, "Why are you always so happy?" or, "No one could be as happy as you!" I became, and still am, always "super". I now realized that the books I was reading had a large influence on me and had caused me to become a positive thinker.

I also noticed I was able to handle my difficult situations and every day irritations better because my thoughts were geared toward problem solution instead of problem worrying. Through reading positive books I learned that most problems can be solved in some way. Solution means the problem is no longer a time-consuming worry. Instead an answer can be determined that at least reduces your involvement with the problem to inconsequential. I learned that nothing will be solved with worry which only hurts the worrier and offers nothing in return but the worsening of the problem. I learned that making a list of all possibilities for reducing the worry and then seeing which ones are really possible will aim me toward solving the problem causing the worry. I learned that handing over to God those problems for which I could find no good apparent solution helped free me from undue worry.

The positive way of thinking became a part of my everyday demeanor because I learned that unless I applied the material I read to my every day life and allowed it to become habit it would be meaningless.

The second event was when I discovered one of my sons was an alcoholic. I began to notice a change in his behavior when he was in the seventh grade. The fact of alcoholism began to become apparent with his first driving while intoxicated (DWI) charge when he was sixteen years old. The judge sent him to a rehabilitation, rehab, center for twenty eight days in an attempt to educate him on the problems with drinking alcohol excessively. He arrived home from those twenty eight days drunk. His school grades, his participation in sports, everything a parent wants for their children suffered immensely. The most suffering though was inflicted on me and my wife.

My son "graduated" from high school, quotes around graduated because he actually was just passed through high school. He went to work for a large excavating company. He was doing well and I thought at the time he had matured enough to understand the problems with chronic drinking. Then he received another DWI. He was a good worker, and smart and personable, so his company sent him to another twenty eight day rehab center. He returned from that center and went back to work. Then there was a third DWI. This time he went to jail for thirty days to repay the community for being a danger to other drivers. He came out of jail and returned to work. As I said his employer liked him and he did really good work. Then he was caught drunk on the job. When the company safety officer investigated he found a stash of many empty vodka bottles hidden in the part of the facility my son worked in. My son was fired.

He was living at home so we then had him at home full time where he continued to drink. I sent him to another rehab center. He returned to only continue drinking. He was becoming a real problem through his destruction of household items and his drunken unruliness. I sent him to still another rehab center but his drinking continued. Following the advice of Alcoholics Anonymous I now made him get out of the house. He had no where to go except into the street. When he attempted to break into my house after I had put him out I had him arrested, had my son arrested. He resisted that arrest and tried to fight with the police officer. When he returned from that jail time he seemed "cured". He took a job working for an automotive repair chain. He did extremely well, so much so they transferred him and paid for his move to one of their stores in Florida. Less then six months after he moved he was fired for not coming to work for several weeks because he was continually drunk.

He is still in Florida, still drinking, still going to rehabs there, but not any longer for the most part at my monetary or emotional expense, and he is still working at times. That seemingly will be his life for as long as it may last through the killing effects of alcohol.

Through all of my son's problems I became aware of the needs of people with diseases. During this time I also became aware of the fact that there are some diseases which I can have little control over the outcome of the diseases effects. This allowed me to develop less impact on my emotions. Lessening of emotions does not mean the loss of love or caring, but the recognition that my son's problem was out of my hands. This allowed me to be clearer about the actions I would need to take to handle his problem in a way that was in the best interests for him, my wife and me. In due time and with great difficulty I learned to practice what Alcoholics Anonymous teaches which is "tough love".

More importantly, I became even more aware of the bible verses that show us how God will handle our problems if we will just turn them over to Him. Verses like John 16:33, Jesus has been through life in this world and has not only overcome the world but, from 1John 5:4, He promises to be there with us so that we too can overcome the world. Then there is 1 Peter 5:6-7 with its consoling message that "we don't have to face life fearfully. As humans we will doubt and fear at times but He offers to shoulder that and all of our burdens". Nothing is perhaps more comforting than in Philippians 1:6 which states "Through all the pain, the trials, the sorrow, the adversities of life, God is working something beautiful in our lives".

I have recognized over the years through my religion that Jesus will carry me through the tough times. There is a poem credited to Mary Stevenson that relates how two sets of footprints in the sand become one. This is where we learn that Jesus does carry us through the tough times in our lives. (See the end of this chapter for the full poem.) I really can pray when I do not know what else to do for God to take over and solve the problem for me. It always works at least for my inner peace because I no longer worry about solving that problem and even though the problem may not have been totally solved it relieved me from suffering and worrying about it. Praying and handing the problem over to God helped me to effectively forget the problem and go on with my life.

This part of my now maturing recognition of the help I could get from God and the things I learned from all the positive thinking materials I had read were really paying off.

I repeat, I love my son, will always love my son but he is not going to stop drinking because I love him. I know of nothing else I can do to get him to stop drinking so my life must go on and go on happily.

The third life changing event that was preparing me to better handle the adversity I was to face began in my son-in-laws basement. As a young boy I had enjoyed playing the guitar and listening to country music. As I was deciding what activities I wanted to start in preparation for having an active retirement I decided playing the guitar again was one thing I would like to restart in my life. My other son had taken guitar lessons for several years and he was excellent at playing that instrument as well as many other instruments. My son-in-law had also started playing the guitar and his brother is an accomplished musician. The four of us started to get together in my son-in-laws basement and play, unplugged as they say, one night a week. Eventually we wanted to be more grandiose so we moved to my son-in-laws brother's larger basement where we added a keyboard and amps for an electric guitar. Two others joined us, a drummer who moved his drum set in and another guitarist.

We got to sounding pretty good for a group without much in the way of electronic equipment to enhance our vocals or instrumentals. Then the drummer built a stage in his basement where we moved our once-a-week rehearsal. Even more we began to realize that the camaraderie we had developed was worth more than developing our musical talents.

At the drummer's house we added more equipment and began to get louder with the addition of more amplifiers. Soon it became difficult for the drummer's son to study so we had to think about moving once again. We did, to my basement after I removed several years of stored old furniture, clothes and just plain junk. In my basement, we continued to add equipment that made us, according to some, sound really good. During this time two other people joined us.

Now we were a band of eight getting better with each week's get-together and building an even stronger camaraderie. We decided we had gotten good enough to record some of our music. That led us on a journey to revamp my basement into a full-fledged studio complete with a soundproof, well almost, control room. Most of us pitched in to perform this transition from a basement band to a basement band with studio. The transformation used many of our combined talents. Each of us really looks forward to our once a week get-togethers, not only for the music but even more the strength of the friendships. The band has become a part of each of our lives but for me it has become something bigger.

These close friends have adopted me as their surrogate Dad and I have adopted them as my surrogate sons. Of course, one is my son, one is my son-in-law and one other is his brother. It is great having them in my life. Whenever life's troubling events, particularly with my wife's illness, would lay me low and bring on sadness one or more of them are always there to brighten my way. When my wife passed away, four days before Christmas, every one of those guys were at my house to be with my son and me. They didn't just come by for a few minutes. They were there for several hours and knowing how most of us guys are I am sure most of them still had a lot of Christmas shopping to finish. On the day my wife was buried, Christmas Eve, the guys and their wives did everything to prepare for the reception at my house following the burial including purchasing the food.

My wife and I always loved Labrador Retrievers (Lab) and usually had one or more to enjoy. When my wife was diagnosed with Alzheimer's we did not have a dog so I decided having a Lab again may help her. It would at least put some additional brightness in her day and in mine. So I bought a six-week-old male black Lab puppy and we named him Bear. (You have seen Billie Jean with Bear in the picture at the beginning of this book.) When I was younger I taught dog obedience classes so now I was able to spend useful time training our new puppy. This also gave me some added activity to help use some time when I was confined to home due to my wife's illness.

Getting this puppy was the fourth thing I had to help me stay happy through one of the saddest events I can imagine. The Lab immediately became a part of the family and was always accompanying one or both of us.

I have often heard how therapeutic animals can be but none could have experienced that more than me. He was also good therapy for my wife. When we would visit our farm in West Virginia and I was doing farm chores our dog would stay with her lying at her feet, helping her to feel secure and less alone. After my wife entered an assisted living facility that characteristic also became some of his contributions to me, helping me feel secure and less alone. He adopted me as his companion. I adopted him as my "Buddy dog" and a friend that I could talk to and complain to and cry to. He listened with a cocked head and provided a loving lick to the chin. When we visited my wife after she entered the assisted living facility the first thing "her" dog would do is put his front paws in her lap and give her a great big "kiss".

For me, going to bed at night with the secure feeling that I was being protected, waking up in the morning to his tail-wagging expression of love, going through the day with a living, breathing being around that I could talk to helped me get through at lot of tough times.

So these four events of learning how to become a positive thinker, having an alcoholic son, a very close group of family members and friends, and getting a Lab that collectively entered my life over the past twenty five years and had no apparent relationship other than they were each a separate and discrete part of my life have combined to become the rock that provided me the means to endure the growing hardship of my wife's progressive succumbing to Alzheimer's.

There is no way I could have known when each of these events occurred that they were preparation for some future event. They were each distinct and different. They were each, except one, a happy event. They were each disassociated. They each started and lasted over a period of years. The most important thing is the consequence of each lasted over the period of time I needed them to help me handle the day-to-day coping required to care for my wife. They continue today helping me cope with the loss of my wife after the many years of dealing with her disease.

So my recognition of the spiritual help needed to help sustain us through adversity is very apparent in my life. Today I realize that my alcoholic son, who says he really does enjoy drinking, was given to me not only because I still love him and have not abandoned him but also to help prepare me for an even greater challenge to lovingly and thoughtfully care for his Mother while maintaining a healthy, enjoyable life for me.

That's where the friendships given to me several years ago come in. Playing music gives me something to look forward to on a weekly basis. Even more, I look forward to being with people whom I truly love and who truly love me. They offer me a sounding board for problems and ideas, they offer a shoulder to cry on, and they offer to help me do chores even if they have their own chores to do.

And my Lab is a daily comfort, sitting and lying by my chair, nudging me for a pat on the head or a scratch behind the ear or even more a scratch at the base of his tail. He is truly my "buddy dog!"

The other significant event that has roots embedded in helping me cope was my involvement in the process of "brain washing" my psyche to become positive in its thinking. I really believe becoming a positive thinker helped me learn to handle life's challenges in a positive and spiritual way.

I believe God is also working in your life. Some of you may not see that now. You may be wondering why God did such and such to you. You may be asking, "Why me God?" You may be denying God's existence because of some hardship you have suffered like having an alcoholic child or a loved one with Alzheimer's.

According to Harold Kushner in his book *When Bad Things*

Happen to Good People, we have to try to rise beyond the question of, "Why did something bad happen to us?" and begin to ask the question, "What do I do now that it has happened?" From my experiences I believe there is no better advice to get us started on the road to handling any adversity in a meaningful and useful manner.

I certainly hope my on-going recovery from coping with my wife's Alzheimer's signals the end to the most tragic event in my life but if not, I am even better prepared to handle adversity in the future.

"Footprints in the Sand" by Mary Stevenson

One night I dreamed I was walking along the beach with the Lord.
Many scenes from my life flashed across the sky.
In each scene I noticed footprints in the sand.
Sometimes there were two sets of footprints, other times there was one only.
This bothered me because I noticed that during the low periods of my life, when I was suffering from anguish, sorrow or defeat, I could see only one set of footprints, so I said to the Lord, "You promised me Lord, that if I followed you, you would walk with me always.
But I have noticed that during the most trying periods of my life there has only been one set of footprints in the sand.
Why, when I needed you most, have you not been there for me?"
The Lord replied,
"The years when you have seen only one set of footprints, my child, is when I carried you."

C 1984 by Mary Stevenson
(see web site http://www.footprints-inthe-sand.com/)

Chapter 3
The Power of Positive Thinking

I have said that learning how to use the power of positive thinking helped me tremendously in meeting all the challenges presented by my wife's disease. Just what is the power of positive thinking?

Let me first define some of life's negative situations the effects of which I have found positive thinking can help reduce if not eliminate. I suspect the most destructive negative trait any person can have is worry. Worry is always a negative in anyone's life. Henry Ward Beecher is quoted as saying, "It is not work that kills people, it is worry. Worry is rust upon the blade." Worry comes in many forms and can be fleeting or consume our entire being for months at a time. Some worry is caused from imagining something may happen without that thing or event ever actually occurring. Worry can manifest itself so deeply in our being that we need to seek professional help to prevent our death either from physical deterioration or self destruction.

When you find yourself starting to worry about something,

starting to have some slight panic about something happening or not happening, the first thing you need to do is determine what you perceive the problem or problems to be that may be causing you to worry, then determine all the potential causes of the problem or problems and then consider all the eventual consequences if the cause of the problem or problems is not greatly reduced or eliminated. Write these things on a piece of paper.

Now consider the worst of the consequences if the problem is not solved. Ask yourself if that occurring will really be so bad. Consequences can range from the trivial to your death. Now ask yourself what all the possible solutions are to the potential causes of the problem. The solutions will be determined by what is needed to reduce or eliminate some or all of the causes thereby avoiding the consequence. Try to come up with as many solutions as you can. Again, write all of this on a piece of paper. Now examine the solutions. Which is the easiest to implement? Will that sufficiently solve the problem? If not, what is the next solution? Will that sufficiently solve the problem? Keep this exercise going for each potential solution until you find one that will sufficiently eliminate the problem. Will some combination of solutions work or work better? Examine that as a possibility.

Can you now solve the problem, that is reduce the cause to satisfactorily allow the problem to be handled? If so, you are done except to implement your solution. If not, go to the second worse consequence of the problem and repeat what you did for the worst consequence. Can the problem now be solved? Continue this for each of the causes, if multiple causes, and for each of the consequences. Most worry causing problems can be solved in this manner.

I went through this process many times. Before learning this technique for handling problems I often found myself in a frenzied state of mind, so much so I was in no way able to solve any problem. After I learned this technique here is a simple example I went through when I experienced some chest pain following one of my wife's visits to the doctor. The pain had been returning for several days and seemed to be getting worse. It even seemed to be causing difficulty breathing. I became worried and even imagined I was having severe heart problems. What did I do? Well, first I tried to think of everything conceivable that could be causing the problem. It could be indigestion, it could be angina, it could be a cracked rib or it could be the beginning of a heart attack. What are the consequences? Well, the worst would result from a heart attack and that could mean death. What needs to be done to solve this consequence? Call my doctor now! But my heart is in good condition. I recently had my annual physical and everything was good. My blood pressure was good, the EKG was good so it really cannot be a heart attack or angina.

The consequences of indigestion can mean loss of sleep, continuing discomfort and eventually perhaps major digestive trouble. My solution is, again, see a doctor, but the physical I had included a follow-up gastrointestinal examination and all was well. In addition, I mostly eat healthy foods and little that could cause prolonged indigestion.

The consequences of a broken rib could mean a punctured lung and the need for an x-ray. Could a broken rib be my problem? Well, four days prior to this while working in the yard I tripped and fell onto some bricks around a flower border. I had forgotten that fall but now in going through this process I recalled the fall and thought a broken rib could be the problem. Now a call to the doctor and an appointment with a radiologist showed indeed I had a broken rib. Whew, and the worry about a heart attack was really beginning to get me down. Boy, did I feel better! Problem solved and no more worry about it. I will also be much more careful when I am occupied with yard work.

Now, you go through this process for each of the things you have that are causing worries you have right now, if any. If no worries now remember this process and use it as soon as some worry begins to consume your thoughts. Not only will this usually find adequate answers to your problems it will also get your mind off of the worry. You are spending your time looking for the means to get rid of the worry, finding the solution to the problem, instead of spending that time worrying about the problem.

Positive thinking enters worry elimination by letting you know that there is usually a solution at least to the extent the problem will be reduced to inconsequential. Even if you are not able to find a solution to the problem, there was none I could find for my alcoholic son, positive thinking allows you to handle that consequence and to move on, continuing to look for solutions but realizing there is nothing more you can do at the time. Actually as I mentioned previously there is another solution I found. That is to turn the unsolvable problem over to God. My prayer about my son went something like this, "Dear God, I have tried and cannot find a solution to my son's addiction and I see no way I can handle it without your help so please lift that problem from me and solve it in your way according to your will. Thank you! Amen!" While not forgetting the problem neither did I worry about it any longer. In fact, as I said earlier, my son was transferred to Florida so I was not any longer directly involved in his life. Do you think this was God's answer to my prayer? I do!

There are some dire problems which have no permanent solution. Alzheimer's is one. In those cases if you are diagnosed with Alzheimer's or any other life taking disease you need to recognize the end result, the consequence and make the best of your remaining life by reducing as much as possible the worry that will manifest itself in many ways. Keeping busy, doing useful tasks are ways to at least temporarily get the worry off of your mind. Keep occupying your mind in any way you can, preferably doing anything that is enjoyable for you. For example, my wife turned her attention to doing needlework. That constantly occupied her until she was not able to work the needles any longer. She made some beautiful things all of which are now a treasure to my children and me. Her prayers for God to handle her problem and to help others may well have resulted in Him giving me the notion to attempt this book and to help others better handle the worry of having Alzheimer's or any other life taking disease. This book is a means of having my wife's long battle with Alzheimer's bring positive results to others. This illustrates the very good effects of how positive thinking can apply to the person suffering from a disease as well as others affected by their loved ones suffering.

How do you handle life's obstacles thrown in your path? How do you get the most out of life? Positive thinking can help in our day to day work and play to make life better or at least seem better. Seem better because if something is happening to us but does not affect the senses of touch, see, smell, hear or taste then the mind is the only other thing most of us have that affects our life through perception and remembered or installed training.

Our mental age is not measured by our years of life but rather by our maturity, by what we have learned and retained, that's installed training. Some people at the age of thirty have the same retained installed training, maturity, which others have not attained at age sixty or more. Then again, some thirty year olds have advanced to the age of sixty in their mental outlook on their life. The point is chronological age is not very important to our mental state. What is important is how you cope with your ongoing life events no matter what your age.

One way I keep active and feeling young is to install in my psyche that I am only twenty five years old. When I am asked my age I will always say, "I'm twenty five!" I am convinced this has a huge effect on my ability to continue to keep up with my much younger friends when we are doing any physical activity. Of course, the activity also has a large and positive effect on my physical ability and appearance.

One primary difference in our maturity is how each of us handles life's adversities. It is not usually your five senses that have much to do with the determination of how you handle obstacles. Well, that's not true if you pick up a hot coal from the grill or the likes but it's your mind that can keep you young or let you age faster than your years. It's your mind that you let get out of control with worry, depression, erroneous thoughts. It's our mind we have to train to handle life's adversities so we can handle those adversities as best we can but at the same time let our mind work to also keeping us focused on getting the most out of life in any situation. This is a focus we all need to get. Don't use "I can't" or anything else as a cop-out to avoid taking the necessary steps to improve your life regardless of your life's progression to where you are now.

Here are some tips I use to train my mind. First, don't settle down into the woe-is-me way of thinking due to some obstacle thrown at you. This can cause you to settle down into a vegetative way of life and that becomes a killer. Unfortunately many people, I have read most but I hope not, merely exist and do nothing but eat, drink and sleep albeit probably not too well. That is no way to be in condition for anything but particularly not a condition that will allow problem solution for problems that will create much worry. Get out of that rocking chair; for goodness sake stay away from that bottle of alcohol; concentrate on broadening your interests; keep up with what is happening near to you and far away; busy yourself with hobbies, home improvement projects, anything that provides entertainment and enjoyment and occupies your mind and body. Choosing some combination in these categories is even better.

In addition to the band and my home gardening projects and my farm, photography has become a hobby for me. With the digital world of today, photography has become a real enjoyment not only in learning the technological processes involved but in the collection of photos I can archive for years of reflecting on various people and past events.

Is there something you have wanted to do and just not taken the time to get started? Getting started is the first big step toward accomplishing whatever it is you want to do. Is there something you did as a youth and now want to continue?

If so, get started. One of mine was playing the guitar and you have already read how that blossomed into a real joy for me and a necessary part of my life.

Another thing I have learned is that regardless of any previous failed starts on some activity I wanted to accomplish I can always restart to achieve a new and beneficial end.

Try to learn at least one new thing a day and then see if you can use it toward something beneficial to you or others. Some of learning new things can come from reading books, circulars, anything that requires you to use your brain. This keeps your brain active and healthy so you are better able to use healthy reasoning to solve those daunting problems. I pat myself on the back each day I have learned something new. I have been heard many times to say, "I didn't know that. I have learned my new thing today!"

Commit yourself to working one crossword puzzle each day to keep your mind active. I get my puzzle completed shortly after getting out of bed in the morning. That also helps to wake up my mind early in the day so it will operate at peak efficiency from the start of the day.

Maybe you have wanted to learn a new trade, a new profession or just learn more about something that interests you. Go back to school. Most communities have educational facilities nearby that offer short, non-credit courses in self improvement or the arts. Many also offer courses toward a degree or an associate degree in many subjects. You are never too old to go back to school. I am sure you, as I, have read the very interesting stories of people in their seventies and eighties who have earned college degrees. Why not you if you do not have a college degree or want another degree in some other field of study? Going back to school will also get you out of the house and with people. Meeting people, being with people is one of the best therapies I know for handling depression and many other negative emotions.

In the past, I have taken several courses just to spend some time learning something new and meeting new people. One course, business law, has helped me in several of my business endeavors. I took a course in getting my real estate license, not because I wanted to become a realtor but because I thought it would give me some insights to real estate investing. Since I started writing this book I took a course on how to get a book published. Through that course and my experience I sure found out it is not an easy thing to do but I did learn what I needed to do.

Would I like to get another degree? Well, to tell the truth I would but I don't know whether I want to be a doctor or a lawyer and given the years involved to achieve either I'll settle for my current life as the Indian chief who can still chop the wood and then sit around the fire and enjoy life.

Maybe you are in a period of your life where you have a little down time. Take advantage of that by gaining some new knowledge or expanding your knowledge in a field that interests you. These things will distract your negative feelings while at the same time improving your attitude, skills and, potentially, your income.

It does not matter what you want to start doing. Each of us has our own likes and dislikes. Just be sure to get started on one or more of your likes. Make plans for whatever that is and be sure to follow through after you get started. William Jennings Bryan, the lawyer, orator and politician is quoted to have said, "Destiny is no matter of chance, it is a matter of choice. It is not a thing to be waited for, it is a thing to be achieved." What we are, who we are, what we will become are all a matter of choice though there are some who leave that choice to chance, which is their choice. R.E. Shay is quoted to have said, "You can depend on the rabbit's foot if you want but remember it didn't work for the rabbit."

The point in all of this is to keep our minds and bodies active. Active minds and bodies is the best way to also keep them fresh, vibrant and young which allows us to better handle life's adversities.

I have mentioned several ways to keep our minds active. For

some, like those with Alzheimer's or other diseases that limit what can be done the list will be smaller but not zero, perhaps for a long time. Here the choice is really the same as for others, decide what you want to accomplish perhaps in limited time and get busy doing it.

    Do you have an "I can" attitude? If not see if you can develop one. I used to have a sign over the telephone that said, "Say I'll try not I can't." I would point to that sign any time my children said "I can't" reminding them that they may not be able to accomplish the topic right now but with the I can't attitude they would never be able to do it. Many of these conversations were about that night's homework. I explained that believing I can't would make the required activity that much more difficult and there was no way they were not going to do their homework. Saying "I'll try" became the preferred response to me and got my help a lot sooner if there really was a problem with their understanding of what to do.

    All of us form habits, some good and some bad. If you have the habit of saying "I can't" then you will never attempt to learn to do whatever is behind the remark. That is a bad habit.

    I have read that it takes twenty eight days to get rid of a bad habit. I have found it takes at least that and a continued focus on continuing the good habit that is replacing the bad habit well beyond the twenty eight days. I suggest if you use "I can't " to deny trying anything you decide right now to eliminate that phrase from your vocabulary for at least the next twenty eight days and use an "I can" approach to whatever you would have used "I can't " to deny doing. Be careful though. Some of us use "I can't" to really mean I don't want to or I should not do that thing. If that is the case you must examine what it is you do not want to do or should not do. If it's jumping off the cliff in Mexico into the ever changing depth of water below your "I can't" is probably well founded in meaning I don't want to potentially cripple myself for life. If your "I can't" means I don't want to take that first step toward solving a significant problem then erasure of using the "I can't" means to stop fooling yourself. The twenty eight day rule would apply since there has to be some means to get you off of that excuse.

For me, I don't believe I have said I can't for a long time. If I don't want to do something or think doing it would be wrong I just say that. I have found that practicing what I preach about being positive really does work.

To that end, I have found that an "I can" attitude is needed to support and enhance a positive attitude and vice versa. One way to help develop that attitude is to constantly tell yourself "I can". Constantly doing this will begin to brainwash your mind to really believing you can and really believing you can is the first step to achieving anything. Did I say brainwash? But I don't want to be brainwashed you say, that is not a good thing. Oh it's not? How did you learn to do arithmetic, learn to read, write or most anything else? Learning is the daily introduction into our minds of many things. As we continue to go over those things, to repeat those things, to practice those things, they become installed in our brains. The things we learn the best and retain the longest are those things we repeat and practice over and over the most. This is the reason there are homework assignments at all educational levels. Homework causes repetitive use of the thing being learned. That is brainwashing! Most of us raise our children to avoid bad peers. That is because the bad peers have been brainwashed in the wrong direction and through continued association our children will become brainwashed in the same direction. So brainwash is just a term to define what we have learned and retained primarily through repetition of use in our every day life.

Part of the "I can" attitude is to constantly review all the things we need to accomplish knowing some will be difficult and some easier or even easy. For best results to your psyche, take on and accomplish the tough things first. This implies prioritizing every item on the list. Do this by sorting each into one of three categories. The first is must be done or at least started regardless of anything else. The second is needs to be done or started but not immediately and the third is the items that can wait until there is time to address them. Now write these items down in the three lists. Chances are most items in the third list are not important and many will never get addressed. That is unless you address those items first because they are easy leaving the most important items un-addressed. Now there is something that may create a cause for worry!

Be sure you continually update your lists. You, as I do, will find some of the items in list two will eventually end up in list three. Items in list three will seldom get done unless we have completed all of the list one and two items. I have found after using this technique to accomplish needed items first that I no longer have to write things down. My habit has become to spend my time each day first doing those things that must get done and second starting those things that must get at least some attention now. If there is time left over, and most of the time there is, then I do the things I want to do which can include items in the third list. For example, when I have bills due that is a list one item I take care of the first thing in the morning. When I have dirty clothes that need laundering that is a list two item that I will at least partially address at some time during the day by sorting the clothes into piles. They can then be washed at any time later during the day or the next morning. Of course, if I have neglected that item for too long it will then become a list one item to prevent my arrest for nudity.

Do you worry about some things you believe need to be done but are not yet accomplished? Making the suggested list of priorities may help you stop those worries especially when the items fall in the third category. When the items are in the first category you now know your priorities and can determine what you need to do. Getting busy solving the things you really need to solve will help to conquer your worry. You need to start today to solve your worry causing problems. Don't procrastinate and wait to start tomorrow. Remember that today is tomorrow's yesterday. Starting now to solve your problems means you will have become an "I can" person.

Closely associated with "I can" and required for the "I can" to be effective is the "I will". "I will" is the determination that you will start toward solving your problems and meeting your needs, your goals. After getting started you then must continue toward your goal until everything required to meet the goal is complete. Without the "I will" attitude your abilities to accomplish anything will likely fade away into the dark recesses of dead brain cells. "I will" is the "put up or shut up" behind the "I can". Your will is the deciding factor in you achieving anything.

As you get started on accomplishing anything you must follow a plan to reach your final objective. For all except insignificant accomplishments be sure you write that plan on a piece of paper listing the interim dates you need to meet interim objectives which will get you to your final objective. Be sure you stay happy and enthusiastic about everything you must do to attain your objective, your goals. Even if the goal is to care for a loved one and to care for yourself in the care of your loved one you can be enthusiastic in recognizing you are making your loved one more comfortable while at the same time insuring you are staying healthy which also will contribute to your loved ones comfort.

For me, I loved my wife and still love my wife. I miss her terribly and think often of how the two of us would be enjoying the activities I have today many of which she and I planned to enjoy together. But she is gone. I set my number one goal of doing all I knew and learned to make her comfortable and well cared for while she was alive. That was my vowed "I will" and I believe I achieved that goal. Now I have the choice of folding up and dying too or continuing to have a life for myself that I enjoy. I believe God intends the latter.

Much of your life spent after meeting and handling the adversity of losing a loved one is associated with the attitude you have toward setting and meeting your desires, your goals, after your loved one is gone. The "I will" attitude keeps you going, active to achievement of the things in life you need and want for your survival and your happiness. After you lose a loved one you may develop a new pattern of life. You may develop new habits, meet new friends. You may even find a new friend of the opposite sex whom you enjoy doing things with and who enjoys doing things with you. This can be especially beneficial to your enjoyment if you are a person like I am who does not like to go places alone. Here the "I will" becomes enjoyment of a new life, enjoyment of new possessions, blazing new trails, meeting another person and enjoying their company. Most important is the enjoyment of a peace of mind that you and your God have gotten you to where you are and will continue to guide you to a fruitful life until He takes you to be with your loved ones who have gone before you.

So prepare to begin any new journey with the "I will" attitude so the "trip" will be successful at each step along the way.

What do you think of yourself? Do you like yourself? Do you hate yourself? Do you feel what you do is important? The lack of something to feel important about is almost the greatest tragedy a person may have. Do you respect yourself? That is necessary before you will respect others. Do you love yourself? You really need to love yourself before you can really love others. I don't mean to be conceited, to be an egomaniac. I mean to be comfortable with who you are, comfortable in your own skin. To be comfortable with what you do letting others "blow your horn". When you let others blow your horn it will have a far greater significance than if you blow your own horn. I mean to be comfortable with being with others. To be comfortable when getting a fair and honest evaluation of you or something you have done. I mean to taking care of yourself mentally and physically. In chapter six I will go into some of what I do to keep physically fit.

There are seven words I heard and read some time ago that have had a really large and welcome impact on me. Those words are, "You are what you think you are!" If you think you are no good than more than likely you are no good. If you think you are not able to do something than you will not be able to do that thing. If you think you will not live to be a ripe old age you will more than likely not live to be a ripe old age. If you think the boss is lousy and picking on you then you will see most of what he or she does as picking on you. If you think you'll lose at something, you did.

On the other hand, if you believe you are a good person, if you believe life is great and getting better, if you believe you can handle your problems, if you believe you can accomplish whatever your needs and wants then your thinking is positive and you are on the right track to accomplishing the things you need and want to accomplish.

Abraham Lincoln is quoted to have said it this way, "People are about as happy as they make up their minds to be." So if you are not very happy now you need to make up your mind to become happy or become happier in your life. If you believe you need improvement in this part of your life you need to take the necessary steps to create the environment that for you will increase the fun you have in your life, to "make your day" every day.

If I had to point to the one thing that was very beneficial in my mental gyrations of dealing with my wife's disease it would have to be this one sentence, "I am what I believe I am." I believed I could care for my wife and still find enjoyment amid the adversity I was going through. Both my wife and I were better off for this way of thinking.

Some people may try to discourage you in this type of thinking. Don't let them! You have to know you are an original so run your own race. Don't try to be a duplicate of someone else and don't listen to others who want to compare you to others or want you to be something you are not. If you try to be like someone else you can only be second best. Trying to be a copycat will make you a kopykat, a cartoon of what you can be. Just be yourself, be the best "you" you can be. Each and every one of us is unique and special. Realizing this we can all nurture our own specialties while at the same time helping others to nurture their specialties.

You need to find friends who are supportive of you trying to improve your life, friends who want to join you in your endeavor for improvement, friends who have the means to help you in achieving your goals. You may try to help those who are negative and trying to prevent your improvement but if they are not willing to receive your help while supporting your ambitions for improvement then you will have to leave them behind as you advance your enjoyment of your life. My family and friends in the band are always encouraging me saying things like, "You sure have learned to play the bass guitar well in a short time", "You can outdo us in physical things", "You are really a smart person" or "You'll outlive all of us". I also return encouraging remarks to them particularly if I hear one of them saying, "I can't do such and such."

Anything you want to accomplish is mostly achievable by knowing you have the ability or can develop the ability to accomplish it. "Carry the dominating thought of your desire to achieve the subject of any thought with you constantly. See your success, your dream "as if" it has already occurred." It is important to write down a description of what you want to achieve and the associated dates of when you want the endeavor completed. Is there a picture of what your goal is? Then post it in a very conspicuous place where you see it every day. Remember the discussion on brainwashing? My wife learned much of this with me. One day I came home from work and there was a picture of a cruise ship on the refrigerator. When I asked why she simply said it was a picture of our next vacation. Each time I walked by the refrigerator, it was many times a day, that ship seemed to get bigger and to draw me closer. Well, our next vacation was not on that ship but only because there was not enough time to book passage before our next vacation time. The next year we took two vacations, the first being a seven-day cruise and would you believe it was on the same ship as shown in the picture.

Be sure everything you put into your plan to accomplish any goal does not have any negative effects on others. Earning good will is like earning a good name, each is obtained by many good actions but will be lost by only one bad action especially if that action hurts another person. I believe my integrity is the one thing I have complete control of. No one can make me do anything that will negatively affect my integrity and hurting others will reflect negatively on me. Instead of hurting others be there for them to help them. Choose to help them "make their day" while you are making your day. I have found that some of the most rewarding achievements are those that help someone else solve a problem, help them become happier in their life. I said earlier that bringing a smile to the faces of people in the assisted living facility was very rewarding for me.

Accomplishing your goals really is as simple as acting on the fact that you are what you think you are and can achieve whatever you desire to achieve. The only way for you to be defeated is for you to accept defeat. Instead be persistent in achieving your desires. To do otherwise will cause you to fail. And by all means do not procrastinate in getting started. This will bring doom to getting anything accomplished. Persistence is cited as being required to stick with your goals and plans to conclusion. A saying worth printing and mounting in a prominent place goes like this:

"Press on, nothing in the world can take the place of persistence; talent alone will not, nothing is more common than unsuccessful people with talent; genius alone will not, unrewarded genius is almost a proverb; education alone will not, the world is full of educated derelicts. Persistence and determination alone are omnipotent."—a quote by America's thirtieth president, Calvin Coolidge.

You are truly the master of your fate. You are the only person who controls you. Others may attempt to control you. Some may be successful but that is solely because you have allowed that to happen. If there is something you want to do, to accomplish, then it is you and only you who must take the initiative to get started and to follow through to the conclusion you intended when you started. If there is something you do not want to do then it is you and only you who must provide the resistance to deny doing what ever it is.

So what is the power of positive thinking? It is the "I can and I will" attitude you have or will develop to start now, to follow through to completion, doing everything you need to do to meet all the needs and wants you have. It is the realization your worries can be solved if only you will begin to solve them. It is the realization you are what you think you are. For example, if you think you are not very happy then you are not very happy but if you will begin to address that sad state of mind by first knowing you can change and will begin to change by initiating the things you need for you to obtain a happier life then improved happiness is right around the corner.

Many of us have heard the phrase, "If you believe it you can achieve it!" You need to set out to prove that to yourself if you do not currently believe it. Dale Carnegie is quoted to have said, "Remember happiness doesn't depend upon who you are or what you have; it depends solely upon what you think." We all need to follow the quote by Jules Renard in that, "as we understand life less and less means to learn to love life more and more." I did not and do not understand why my wife was chosen to get Alzheimer's but I have learned to enjoy my life by knowing I assured the very best care for her and some such thing as Alzheimer's could happen to me at any time.

This is a story about a man named John I saw on the internet. John can be any positive thinking person. John is always in a good mood and always has something positive to say. When someone asks him how he is doing he replies, "Super, if I were any better I would be twins." John is a natural motivator. If someone is having a bad day, John would tell the person how to look on the positive side of the situation.

One day a friend said to John, "I don't get it. You can't be positive all the time. How do you do it?" John answered, "Each morning I get up I say to myself, "You have two choices, you can choose to be in a good mood or a bad mood today." I always choose to be in a good mood. Each time something bad happens to me I can choose to be a victim or I can choose to learn from it. I choose to learn from it." The friend protested, "But it's not that easy, right?"

John answered, "Yes it is. Life is all about choices. When you cut away all the junk every situation is a choice. You choose how to react to situations, you chose how you let people affect your mood."

There was a time when John was involved in a fall and was seriously injured. After much surgery and weeks of intensive care he was released with rods placed in his back. Soon after this his friend saw him and asked how he was. John's answer was, "Super, if I were any better I'd be twins." The friend protested again saying, "But John, what went through your mind as you lay on the ground seriously wounded?" John replied, "The first thing that went through my mind was the well-being of my soon-to-be-born child. As I lay there I remembered I had two choices, I could choose to live or I could choose to die. I chose to live. When I got to the emergency room I saw in the expressions of the doctors and nurses "he's going to die". I got really scared. I knew I had to take some action. I got the opportunity when a nurse asked if I were allergic to anything. I replied, "Yes, I sure am, I'm allergic to gravity!" After the laughter subsided John told them, "I am choosing to live so operate on me as if I am alive and not as though I am dead." John lived. His friend learned from him that every day presents us with choices and we have to choose to live fully. That is an attitude and after all, attitude is everything.

Positive thinking is an attitude we all need to adopt. It will make many trying circumstances in our lives manageable and for some more quickly solved. I said earlier when I am asked my age I reply, "Twenty five." Sometimes the response to that is, "Twenty five and no hair, huh?" My response is, "Yes, that's right, I'm not old enough to have grown hair yet!" That positive attitude has kept me feeling and acting young, has allowed me to continue to do things that at least I am convinced I could not do if I had the attitude of being much older. I spend each and every day believing that, "Youth is not just a time of life, it is also a state of mind."

Having a positive attitude has been significant in my being able to handle my wife's long struggle with Alzheimer's.

Chapter 4
Legal and Administrative Needs

There are several legal and administrative items that need to be addressed and completed before you or a dependent require significant medical care whether at home, in a hospital, in a care facility or any other place where confinement is due to mental or physical illness. Some items are needed just to be sure you or a dependent are properly represented and your liabilities are covered as you age and when you die. Even if you currently have some or all of what will be covered in this chapter you need to review each item annually and as soon as you or a loved one is diagnosed with a debilitating disease. When my wife was diagnosed with Alzheimer's we reviewed all of our legal documents and important information. That review prompted us to make an appointment with our attorney and make some changes to some of the documents like wills, trusts, health care power's of attorney (HCPOA) and durable powers-of-attorney while she was still legally competent to sign the revised documents.

Items to address include a list of all important types of information and where they can be found if you are unable to tell someone where they are. Your wills, trusts, living will or health care power of attorney (HCPOA), power of attorney or durable power of attorney, insurance policies, investments, personal property listed in an inventory, deeds to real estate and car titles all need to be in a known place and available. If you own guns, the manufacturer, type of gun and gun serial number need to be included with the list of important information. This is information that will be needed not only if the guns are lost or stolen but if you are incapacitated.

Important administrative information includes social security numbers for you, your spouse and children; safe deposit box number and bank where it's located; city and state of birth for you, your spouse and children; parents' names including Mother's maiden name and places and dates of their birth; names, addresses and phone numbers of your doctors, attorneys, investment advisors; accountants; a list of all active credit cards and the credit card number; a listing of all investments by name, type and account number; all insurance policies listing the carrier, the type of insurance and the policy number; summary of real estate investments including location, mortgagee, if any, and type of property, for example rental or second home.

I personally learned the great disadvantage of not having this information available and up-to-date when my Father-in-law's second wife passed away. It became my responsibility to settle her debts and determine the assets and liabilities left in her estate. None of the items and information I have mentioned, including a will, were anywhere to be found and my Father-in law, who was eighty five years old, had not taken any time before his wife's death to locate any information, including her separate debts. So I had to go through her things finding pieces of the information in multiple places. Her social security number, life insurance policies, bank accounts, credit card information all were scattered in various places among many documents. It took over a week spending full time to find and catalog all of her information and I had to make many phone calls to verify what I was finding before I could settle her estate. It didn't help that she had bank statements and other documents from the past several years stuffed in any nook and cranny she could find. Incidentally, I also found over six hundred dollars crammed in envelopes in corners of drawers and in cans hidden in various places.

After putting together her assets and debts I now had to file all the paperwork to get the assets and pay her bills. My Father-in-law had no problem signing whatever was needed to accomplish the task and since there was no will, thank goodness he was able to give the signatures as the surviving spouse.

I was not a hundred percent successful after the first go around. For example, I was sitting in one of the banks with my Father-in-law where his wife kept her accounts closing one of her checking accounts when my Father-in-law pulled some things from his wallet including a credit card with his wife's name. I had previously found no information that alluded to the card. Luckily the card had been issued by the bank we were sitting in so I asked the clerk we were talking with to check the card number to see if there was a balance. There was a six thousand, eight hundred dollar balance. I immediately paid off the debt but then had to write a letter to another organization to close the account.

Also, my Father-in-law's wife had a niece who would show up and rummage through her aunt's things taking whatever she wanted when I was not there. She took jewelry, a one-carat diamond and antique furniture. My Father-in-law did nothing to stop her.

None of these things would have happened if there had been a good, accurate and up-to-date listing of all the information her executor needed to get assets and pay the debts. If she had a will there could have been no pilfering of the assets by anyone except the heirs she named and then only after the will went through probate.

I cannot tell you how much grief I was spared by having all of this important information documented and updated on a regular basis, at least annually, for my wife. There were many occasions during her illness I needed various items of the legal and important information I have mentioned.

There is the need for a safe deposit box to safely store all of this information. You also need to designate another family member or your agent to have access to your safe deposit box if you are not able to access it at the time stored information is needed. The person you designate needs to visit the bank with you and sign the access card to be able to gain entry to the safe deposit box.

Do you have a will? If not then it is now time to get one. According to Consumer Reports seventy percent of American adults do not have a will. Why? Many say it is purely inertia. Most people do not plan to die in the next year. If you die suddenly without a will you will stick your family with an undue burden at a time they do not need more strife. If you have children it is imperative you get a will now if you do not have one. If you have young children they will need a guardian if their parents are lost in an accident and the assets from your estate will be needed to support them in the best possible manner. Without a will the laws of your state will apply and these laws will seldom accommodate your children or your assets in the manner you would want.

You should see an attorney to draw up your will. They know the laws of your state and can be very helpful in making sure all your wishes are documented correctly. If you do not have an attorney call several and get the estimate of their fees. Select one and get your will drawn up.

If you find you cannot afford an attorney's fees there is good information on the internet, in libraries or you can purchase computer software that will help you write a will. Of course, you need to know the laws of your state before attempting this. For example, when my Mother passed away I found at that time the state of Virginia, where she resided, allowed holographic, hand-written, wills which she had. There was no requirement for a witness to the signature. If I had known this before she passed away I could have prevented some later difficulties that arose. Also, these laws can change at any time. Annual updates then need to be done with full knowledge of the current laws in your state. That is a good reason to hire an attorney.

If you have written your own will you will need witnesses to your signature. Depending on your state of residence you will need either two or three witness signatures. These persons will sign your will as witnesses listing their full name and address.

Your will may be modified by you at any time through execution of a codicil to the will. The act of writing a codicil to your will is much easier if you have an attorney write the original will. For me, a phone call to my attorney with the changes I needed was all it took. He first made the changes and mailed me a copy for my review. I phoned him with my approval or changes and he made the final document. I then stopped by his office to sign the document which was witnessed in his office. This all took only a few minutes at minimal cost. If the codicil has been written independent of an attorney, you still need to have your signature witnessed by the two or three witnesses depending on your state.

Wills must go to probate to go into effect after you die. Probate has a cost and is accomplished in the state courts so there are delays, sometimes for long periods of time, in your named heirs getting their proceeds from your estate. Also, wills are public domain so anyone has access to your information.

Revocable trusts are a way to avoid having a will go to probate. They can also help avoid estate taxes depending on your net worth. If you want to avoid probate regardless of your wealth you will need a revocable trust. Revocable trusts are just that, revocable or amendable by the settlor, you, during your lifetime. You are also the trustee of the trust during your life. To get the full tax advantages of a revocable trust requires you to name a trustee other than yourself or your spouse who will manage all the assets named in your trust should you become incapacitated or after you die.

A married couple would set up revocable trusts by deciding which assets, real and personal, are to be placed in each trust with the value split being roughly one half to each trust. It may be necessary to have real property re-deeded to accomplish that split. I had two pieces of deeded real estate held jointly so I had to get both pieces re-deeded with one being in my name and the other in my wife's name.

Be careful who you name as trustee, for both spouse's trust.

I had missed the point that I would not be in total control of my wife's trust when she died because I was not the named trustee. Should your spouse die before you, as in my case, that trust will then become managed by the named trustee. Normally the management will be for the benefit of the surviving spouse but the manipulation of assets in the trust is only accomplished by the approval of the trustee. This could be a real problem if the wrong person is named as the trustee. For the surviving spouse, their trust with all its listed property continues to be controlled by the surviving spouse.

Spouses naming themselves trustees of each others trust can be done but that could undo one of the purposes of setting up revocable trusts, namely the avoidance of paying estate taxes. If each trust names each spouse as the trustee and the combined net worth of your and your deceased spouse's estate exceeds for example two million dollars, then upon the death of the second spouse estate taxes will have to be paid on the excess over two million dollars of the combined assets in each trust. Naming someone other than yourself and your spouse as the trustee of each trust will allow each spouses estate to reach two million dollars before estate taxes have to be paid on either. That number, two million dollars, has only recently grown to be that large and is scheduled to grow to three and one half million dollars but Congress can legislate changes to that at any time so be sure to keep up with changes in estate tax laws if you currently have a revocable trust. Actually your attorney should be the one that keeps up with the changes in the law and notifies you when you are affected. My attorney does and at times may have me come in for a consultation on what the changes mean to me.

After one of a married couple dies, when the surviving spouse passes on their trust will take effect and designate the pay out of that estate to the heirs. Your predeceased spouse's trust also needs to indicate that pay out from that trust to your named heirs will take place upon the death of the second of the couple. These conditions of revocable trusts are covered in the wording, decided by you, of the trust at the time they are initiated.

Revocable trusts require the experience and knowledge of a good estate attorney. When choosing your attorney, as with wills, be sure to obtain estimates for the services needed to obtain a revocable trust. Fees to draw up revocable trusts are usually much higher than drawing up a will. Also, if the attorney is new to you ask for the experience the attorney has in producing revocable trusts. My attorney was recommended by my financial advisor and he is knowledgeable and experienced in all estate needs.

For me, having revocable trusts in force at the time my wife passed away saved a lot of hassles which would have added to my grief. One trip to my attorney assured I would not have to probate my wife's will and there would be no estate taxes since the dollar amount of her trust did not exceed the allowed limit and the trustee of her revocable trust had become the manager of her named assets. These trust assets do not include life insurance policies and retirement plans like IRA's since they pay to the named beneficiary on each of those assets. Of course, if the trust is the named beneficiary then those assets will go to the trust and be managed by the named trustee of the trust.

Having a living will or Health Care Power of Attorney(HCPOA) is also imperative. The HCPOA is different and better than a living will since the HCPOA allows your designated agent to make your health care decisions for you at the time those decisions are needed and based on the information available at that time. A living will or HCPOA is very different from a will. I am sure most of you have heard some of the very sad situations of a loved one being "brain dead" or in a vegetative state and family members quarreling over whether to have life support removed or not. All of that can usually be averted through a living will or HCPOA. These documents are your designation of your desires for you under those life terminating conditions. For example, do you want administration of hydration and nourishment through a tube inserted into your stomach to keep you alive if the doctors say there is no way for you to survive off of those mechanical means of delaying your death? These are the types of designations you make in your living will or HCPOA. My doctor initially told me about HCPOA and suggested I get one. I contacted my attorney and he produced one for me and my wife.

I found some of the wording in my initial HCPOA to be confusing as to what I would or would not get if I became vegetative so I went to my doctor to get explanations. After getting the explanations of what the medical meaning was to several of the items in the HCPOA I was then prepared to make my designations of the care I wanted under those conditions. I did not find the thought processes of determining my HCPOA wishes to be particularly enjoyable but know they were very necessary to relieve my family of the burden if I ever become brain dead. It's never too early to have a HCPOA. The time to make your health care decisions for the future is while you are healthy.

As with other legal documents, it is best to have an attorney draw up your HCPOA. As I said, my attorney produced it including witnessing of my signature in a very short time. There is information on the internet or computer software that can be obtained to write your HCPOA or a living will. Here again you must know the difference between the two documents and know the laws of your state that govern whichever you choose.

Next in the list of legal documents you need is a durable power of attorney. It is called durable because it has staying power in the event of your disability. This document names the agent you desire to perform all of your needs for you as if it were you actually performing them for yourself. Here you also need to name successor agents in case the named agent cannot perform. The durable power of attorney takes effect whenever you are deemed not competent to realistically attend to your affairs while you are alive. Your agent then takes over and executes any and all of your business for you regardless of the nature of that business.

The durable power of attorney I had for my wife, after she became legally incompetent, meant I was able to do everything for her without delay whether it involved finances in her name, real estate in her name, medical decisions for her, signing her into a home, whatever the situation, I was able to perform all items as if she were doing them for herself.

Attorneys prepare durable powers of attorney but as with other attorney prepared documents get estimates before engaging an attorney to prepare the document.

I cannot stress strongly enough the need for these documents before any need for their use occurs. Having these documents eliminates a lot of worry and eases the burden on family members required in most circumstances of disability or death. My wife and I each obtained a will soon after the birth of our first child. We had none of the other documents until I had enough assets to hire a financial advisor. He was the person who told us we needed the remaining documents which we quickly obtained from, as I have said, the attorney suggested by our advisor. My advice to you is not to wait until someone else tells you about these documents. You now have that information and everyone needs a will, a living will or HCPOA and a durable power-of-attorney. Revocable trusts can be more of a choice if you do not have current assets over two million dollars soon to become three and one half million dollars or if you do not care that your estate information will become publicly assessable.

I want to emphasize that enlisting an attorney was a tremendous help to me and to my wife when we initially had these documents drawn up. We received very knowledgeable help in the preparation of wills, HCPOA, durable powers of attorney and revocable trusts. We had no concerns that the laws of our state were being met and that all pertinent details were covered in each document as we wanted them to be documented. Today my attorney follows up with me on any changes to any type of document I need to be aware of. He is also a phone call away when I have any question about changes to any of the documents. He is also very liberal in his fee reductions for continuing work I need to have done. This and other advantages are only available when you maintain the same attorney for all of your estate legal needs. My attorney has surely become, along with my doctor, accountant and financial advisor, a large part of the reason I do not have many of the worries I would have without them.

If you believe you cannot afford an attorney the first thing to do is to contact several for a free estimate of their fees to draw up these documents to meet your desires. If now you know you cannot afford the fees the next thing to do is to see if one will lower their fees. There are attorneys who will lower their fees if they are convinced you are not able to afford their usual and customary fees.

If you are persistent in not using an attorney then use the internet to get your information or go to the library for texts on the subjects or purchase software for your computer. Another way to get the information is to look at someone else's prepared documents and make the changes you need for your documents. One thing you will usually need for all of these documents regardless of where the information came from are the witnesses to your signature and, for some, notaries for the signatures.

My Father-in-law had reached the age of eighty five and had none of these documents. I knew he would not take the initiative to get them since he and many others like him had not taken the time to get the documents prepared in the past. Neither would he see the expense as necessary. My Father-in-law had survived two wives, prostate surgery and was now preparing to sell his home and most of his personal property and enter an independent living facility with assisted care as he may require at a future date. He was also getting forgetful so it was becoming apparent he would eventually reach the point of being unable to handle his affairs or to care for himself. I told him it would be in his interest to let me help him get the legal documents he needed. He agreed but as I predicted he would not take the time or allow the expense to go to an attorney. I then went to my documents that I have for the items he would need; a will, a durable power of attorney and a HCPOA. I modified these documents to fit my Father-in-law's situation. I then arranged a meeting with him and three other unrelated persons as witnesses to sign the documents. Did that ever turn out to be a blessing for me and for him. Later I became his caregiver and with these documents I was able to help him on a lot of things he could not do for himself.

With the durable power of attorney I had the ability to cancel credit cards, to get him treated by doctors and to have him admitted to a nursing home. When he ended up in the end condition to his life in a hospital I was able to produce a valid HCPOA so the hospital had his wishes for life support first hand. When he passed away I did not have to probate the will since I had been named on several of his assets like the checking account but mainly since his daughter, my wife, was his sole beneficiary. This was only true though because I had durable power of attorney for my wife who was incapacitated with Alzheimer's and in an assisted living facility at the time of her Dad's death. You will not be as fortunate as I was unless you insist that these documents are completed and reviewed annually for any family member who does not have them.

As an aside here, I did not tell my wife her dad had passed away. I said earlier that I was never sure what may be registering somewhere back in the recesses of her brain. I could not imagine her understanding her dad was gone and she not being able to express her resultant emotion. I would not tell you this decision on my part was correct or not correct but I did everything in my power to not hurt my wife or to cause her any undue grief even though in the later stages of Alzheimer's she displayed little reaction to these types of things. You will need to make the same type of decisions for your loved one if you are the care giver.

My wife and I learned of the need for a home inventory from friends we knew years ago. They were insurance agents who told us of the very sorrowful situations they had seen when all of an individual's or families possessions were lost through catastrophes of fire or natural disaster and no home inventory was available. If you have not heard of the need for a home inventory I hope the next few paragraphs will become your "friend".

A home inventory of personal effects is required by insurance companies as proof of ownership and item value for maximum recovery of assets after the loss in a fire or some natural disaster. Be sure to list each item you own and the original cost. If you have antiques, art, jewelry or other such items of value, they may not be covered under your homeowner's insurance so you will need to get an appraiser to assess their value. That value needs to then potentially be insured under a separate personal property policy if the total value exceeds coverage under your homeowner's or renter's policy.

Having a home inventory is also very important in helping to settle your estate after you pass away. The value of the items will be needed to help settle your estate tax liabilities. The home inventory and the value of each item is also needed when you go through the inventory with your children to pre-determine who gets what after you and your spouse are gone. Be sure to put each child's name by the item they get so there is no question after you are both gone. Children are usually under a lot of stress at the loss of their last parent and may not be in a condition to think straight about the dividing of property. Later this could result in a rift between some or all of the children. Children are usually upset at the loss of either parent. I make the point of last parent because normally all assets pass to the surviving spouse of a married couple. It's the death of the last surviving parent that will normally provide for the division of the estate to surviving children and grandchildren. This predetermining the distribution of assets can usually prevent a rift between siblings, a rift that does not need to occur if the distribution is agreed to with them while you are alive. Of course there is nothing wrong with distributing some assets to your children after the death of the first spouse.

I developed the list of my assets to be divided among my children by escorting them, together, through each room in the house. As the determination was made, by them, as to who wanted what I noted who was to receive it. That completed inventory list with who receives what it is a part of my revocable trust.

One last piece of advice on home inventories. If you or a family member or friend have a video camera take a video close-up of each item in each room. Narrate the video including the person designated to receive the item. This is further protection of your assets for maximum insurance collection from a loss while you are alive and leaves less for interpretation after you are gone. I particularly enjoyed narrating the video of my assets. It let me show off some of the "ham" in me as I was describing each item. For example, I described the old antique grandfather's clock as, "A relic that has lost both its tick and it's tock but by looking at it anyone can still see it's a clock. This item goes to my daughter."

Once you have all of the documents you need they need to be stored in your safe deposit box as well as having a copy of the legal documents left with your attorney, another good reason for having an attorney.

Having all the required documents means you'll have fewer worries as a care giver for your ailing loved one with the knowledge you know their wishes and will be able to perform their wishes as they desired. Also, your wishes will be handled as described in the required documents after you pass on. Your surviving children and in some cases grandchildren will also appreciate the ease of transition of all their parents' and grandparent's assets to them when these documents exist and are up to date.

Chapter 5
Building and Protecting Your Assets

You may wonder what building your assets has to do with you caring for a loved one with Alzheimer's or other diseases whether you are a family member or the main caregiver. The answer is a lot.

When you are getting started in life with your first job that you intend to sustain you and perhaps a spouse later unless you are already married, your thoughts will be on now, the present, when it comes to spending your income. There is the cost of food, lodging, entertainment, credit cards and the like. If you are already married those costs are close to doubled. There is little thought on the part of most young folks and many middle aged folks about the future but it is thinking about the future everyone needs to spend some time on particularly when it comes to building your assets. The debt many people develop regardless of age is mostly due to thinking primarily about the wants, not the needs, for now. This most of the time occurs without any thought about delayed gratification which can actually make the purchase of whatever you want much more appreciated than if you spend now and incur a large debt.

Early in my life I had wanted a new car, actually a Ford T-bird convertible. I had a used four-door Chevrolet. My need was to have transportation which was completely satisfied by the Chevy. I delayed getting a new car until I had graduated from college and was working in my first job after college. Then I could afford a new car so I bought a brand new bright shiny red and white Buick LeSabre sport coupe. My wife and I now had the time to spend doing a little traveling. We felt like the king and queen as we tooled around in that car and we knew we were not being financially drained which increased the enjoyment. Delayed gratification really paid off for us.

If you have gotten in a high debt position you have probably used credit cards to support your erroneous passion for spending without regard for delayed gratification. That means you now have to go through some debt elimination process all the while giving some other organization lots of your money in the form of interest and perhaps late pay penalties simply because you were not willing to wait to get the desired item. There are many people who use credit cards that end up with large stressful debt problems. If you are in that category than I strongly suggest you use the problem solution techniques of chapter three to form a plan to eliminate most of your debt now. I can assure you the benefits based on my experience will be tremendous both to your financial as well as, for most, your mental well-being.

So thinking about the future regarding your finances is required. This thinking about the future is not a requirement limited to young people. It is needed by everyone until retirement and then some. My point in mentioning young people is that is where thinking and planning for the financial future is best started but if you are middle aged or older and have not done such thinking then the following is equally important for you. For example, if a dollar is invested at some percent for thirty years then it will have grown to a much larger value than if it had been invested for twenty years or less at the same percent but will grow to nothing if nothing was ever invested.

I was fortunate in recognizing early in life that the interest I paid to lending institutions was a large added cost to whatever I bought, particularly as it applied to credit cards. The interest on most credit cards is huge, usually two to three times the interest on most mortgages and car loans. Both, mortgages and car loans are needed by most of us who buy a home or a car for needed transportation. These loans fall into the category of things we need. That is seldom true for all the charges many people put on credit on a monthly basis. As I received my monthly statements from credit debt I would look at the amount of interest being charged. It was not difficult to see the large amount of added money I was paying and many of the items purchased were not in any way needed at that time. My wife and I both decided that given our circumstances, we started with nothing but the clothes we owned and I was still in school and paying all costs associated with that, we would not charge anything else unless it was absolutely needed. We found our credit debt was greatly reduced and we actually got to the point each month where we had some money left over after paying the rent and other necessary expenses. We also decided that saving that money would now put interest in our pockets instead of having it taken out of our pockets through interest paid to the credit issuing companies. We opened a savings account and that was our first introduction to watching the number of dollars we owned grow instead of decreasing each month. We also found we did not miss the items we were not buying. Actually, we got a lot more positive jolt at seeing the accumulation of assets in our favor. Mind you, our assets were not growing at a record setting pace but the numbers were getting bigger each month. Though far from being wealthy we began to feel like we were wealthy. What a great feeling!

I believe the most common excuse I have heard for not investing something of one's assets is, "I cannot afford it." My response is, "You cannot afford not to invest." I know most of you have heard the old adage of saving ten percent of your earnings. That is a very good goal to set and to achieve. It is only a dime out of a dollar, ten dollars out of a hundred. This amount will be achievable if you think it can be achievable. Think it, believe it and it will happen. I think you have read that somewhere before! You, as my wife and I did, may have to give up something from your current manner of spending to make it happen but I can tell you from the experience we had in giving up all but needed credit debt that giving up some expenses is well worth doing. For instance, some of the things to consider giving up are, first, smoking if you are a smoker. Not only will you save a lot of money now but you will save more later when the perils of tar and nicotine and the other gasses in tobacco catch up to you by damaging your health. I am an ex-smoker. After smoking for thirty years I know something about what it takes to stop and every bit of that is worth it many times over from a health and monetary standpoint.

Consider going to one less movie a month, buy one less six pack a week, or have one less meal out a week. Do you rent several movies each week? Consider fewer rentals and instead pick up a good book from the library. (How about getting one of the books I have referenced in the appendix?)

Notice I did not say stop all of your discretionary spending. My wife and I still went to the movies, still ate out on occasion but we were now in control of what we earned and what we spent to allow for a break-even or gain in our assets and not a loss each month. We all need some amount of enjoyment that results in a break from our otherwise busy lives. Just be careful to control that spending using some of the thoughts I have offered.

Before spending anything to support your material wants ask yourself, "Do I or do we really need another gadget now?" Learn to say "no" when the item is not meeting a need and you will have to borrow to obtain it. Impulse buying causes many people a lot of grief. Grief in the form of continuing payments that many times will out last the item bought. Learn now to practice delayed gratification. I have said how this added to the enjoyment of my purchases like that shiny new Buick because I had wanted the item for a while and also because I could now afford the item. Notice the word "afford." It is not always the case you must be able to pay all cash for any item you want. You just have to be able to afford it. As an example, it you want something that costs one thousand dollars and you have to finance all one thousand dollars and that cost plus interest will create a larger debt then you can afford then you will have to delay the purchase until you have saved at least some of the total amount and can afford to finance the balance. Saving toward purchasing that item could then mean, if you still even want the item after some time passes, you may be able to buy it outright but for sure you only have to finance an affordable fraction of the total cost still leaving money left in your pocket for other things like investing in your future.

If you do not believe any of this can work for you, you just have too many expenses and work two jobs or whatever the excuse then at least save the pocket change you have at the end of each day. Put that change in a savings account each week. That will add up and allow you to start some investing toward your future.

When you start investing what should you invest in? If you have few assets then a place to start is a bank savings account, a certificate of deposit(CD) or a money market fund. My wife and I opened a bank savings account. These do not usually pay as much interest as some other investments but they do pay some interest so you now have some assets that are working for you even while you sleep. That's right, investments work for you. Instead of you spending more time on the job, working a second job or whatever you may do for added income, your investments work for you full time, twenty four/seven in today's lingo. Your investments earn money for you without you doing one thing except go to the bank or mail that investment check on whatever frequency you decide but I suggest no longer than once a month. My investments are working for me every day during my retirement instead of me having to continue to work during my golden years. Several times a year I get a check from my investments for enough money to more then double my total retirement income from a pension and social security and still leave enough in the investments for them to continue to grow. That good feeling I had when my wife and I first started to see our assets grow just got a lot better.

Does your employer offer a 401k plan? Many do and more are adopting that way of helping their employees save for retirement. Many of those employers also will match some percent of employee contributions to the plan. That is added money to your savings that everyone who has the opportunity needs to take full advantage of.

Your investments need to be difficult to withdraw so I suggest you decline a checking privilege with your savings and investment accounts. A single bank checking account will normally be sufficient for you to mail funds to pay your bills or make purchases in stores. Many banks today offer free checking accounts for maintaining some minimum level of balance. An automatic deposit to a checking account will also get you free checking at many banks today.

As you watch your assets grow through appreciation, dividends and interest, whether it's a dollar growth a week or one hundred dollars a week or more, most people will be encouraged to invest even more. Just getting started is the hurdle you have to get over. Have you read that somewhere before?

Some of you have enough to invest now. Maybe your income has grown to exceed your needs, maybe you have been saving and have a nice nest egg already started. Then where you invest those assets becomes the decision you have to make. If you are still young, middle aged or entering your senior years investing to maximize the growth of your assets and to maximize the income from those assets is your goal. The method you need to implement to achieve this goal is diversification, investment in a varied number of different investment vehicles to maximize gain and lower the risk of loss over the long term. This is where for example mutual funds, bonds, real estate investments and treasury notes all come into play. My assets are in many of the different types of investment vehicles available.

Should you continue to make these investment decisions for yourself as you did when perhaps you started out with saving your pocket change? The answer, I believe, is "no" unless you are a Certified Financial Planner (CFP), currently engage a CFP or have similar and continuous training in all types of investments and how to read the various market conditions and directions. Certified Financial Planners are folks that go to school to learn the very complicated intricacies of various investment vehicles and the interactions of those vehicles so they can recommend to you an assortment of all those that best fit your investment needs and wishes for the future including your retirement. Taking into account your wishes, goals, is very important. For example, some people want to travel, some want to purchase a second home in the mountains or an ocean front second home or both, some want to just be able to enjoy a comfortable home with a few nights out a week.

How much money do you need to reach your goals? Certified Financial Planners will determine that and put together an investment plan for you based on your current assets, current income and your goals.

Early in life I decided to set a goal to retire at the age of fifty five so my wife and I could enjoy our life together after raising our children. I set that goal and started investing to achieve it. As you now know the financial goal was achieved but enjoyment of a life together with my wife after retirement was not achievable. Substantial assets we had saved now had to be used to care for my wife instead of the two of us using them together for our enjoyment.

I said at the beginning of this chapter that building assets is very important to be able to meet the financial needs of the family and caregiver of someone with Alzheimer's or any other debilitating disease. The financial goal I had set earlier which initially had nothing to do with caring for my wife, allowed me to now accomplish two things financially: First to provide the assets needed to care for her and second to have enough left over for me to enjoy the rest of my life at the life style I am accustomed to. These two things would not have happened without earlier in my life initially recognizing the advantages of saving toward a goal. Now with my assets still growing and the help of a CFP I developed a new strategy for investing that could achieve my changed goals to include caring for my wife. So you can see that building assets initially for one goal was very necessary for me to meet the changed goal of caring for my wife. When I started saving I had no idea what-so-ever the even greater benefit I and my wife would receive was to be able to keep her well cared for during her long illness.

The fact I started fairly early in life and followed through had something to do with my changed goal achievement. That is not to say that whatever your financial status is at the present time or whatever your age, if you have not saved much, beginning now to save or increase your current savings can help you in your future. Even if you never have to care for a sick loved one, one day your paycheck will stop. You have to plan for that occurrence starting now regardless of your age. When you reach that plateau in your life it needs to be a happy occasion, not a sad one, but you will have to live on what's left after the paycheck stops so start planning now to finance a happy retirement. I can assure you it is well worth it.

Most Certified Financial Planners are very good at working with you to help achieve your goals. Some though are not so be sure to get several references from a few CFPs before you pick your planner. The fees from various planners also vary so know those fees up front and what they will do for you with those fees.

Most Certified Financial Planners not only will recommend and handle your investments, they will also suggest what insurance coverage you need for each of the conditions you need to have insurance. This includes life insurance and long term care insurance. When you have one agent for insurance needs and your investments then that person can help you sort through the balance of each as you age and your needs for various insurance types and investments increase or decrease.

For example, I learned not to keep or acquire whole life insurance policies or any other form of permanent life insurance that combines some form of investing along with the death coverage. These two things, investing and insuring, I believe need to be managed separately and not combined in the same vehicle like most whole life policies. The cost of whole life insurance is usually much more than plain term life insurance and the savings you accrue in whole life policies is normally less than you can earn through other investments. Certified Financial Planners will show you that difference and usually recommend term life insurance, normally the least expensive life insurance. You need to buy term life insurance that will cover your financial obligations should you die. There is usually a changing need for life insurance over time. As you grow older that need typically declines since for example, children are grown, college tuitions have been paid, the house is or almost is paid for. These changing needs are usually better covered through term life insurance. Take the amount saved by not purchasing a whole life policy and use it for the long term care insurance you need or add it to the funds you will invest. That way you control the amount of life insurance you need and you control your investing as two separate items. Any good CFP can handle all of these transactions.

I initially had whole life insurance policies which I continued to purchase as our children were born and as we purchased our first home. I kept these policies and paid large premiums until I learned through my first CFP what I have covered here. I converted all of those whole life policies to term insurance in the amount I needed at the time I converted. I might add I got letters from the insurance carriers attempting to dissuade my actions but I was not concerned. I was still covered with the dollar amount of life insurance my family would need if I died. The left over assets from the greatly reduced premiums were invested in things that grew significantly larger in assets than the amounts paid through the more expensive whole life policies I had. In addition, as my need for life insurance declined I reduced the amount of my term coverage on the policy renewal dates until today I carry five thousand dollars worth of life insurance and that is given to me by the company from which I retired. I have used the money saved to purchase more investments and for helping to pay long term care insurance premiums.

You must remember that you have to die for someone else to collect your life insurance so unless you have obligations you want to assure are paid after you are dead you do not need life insurance. It will do YOU no good.

There is an investment vehicle usually sold by insurance companies that has an investment benefit but is not insurance. It is an annuity. Annuities generally have a maturity clause and will pay you under several options chosen by you so if you purchase an annuity be sure you understand the terms of pay out. Incidentally, these pay outs occur while you are alive so unlike life insurance you do not have to die for someone else to benefit from your purchase. As a means of diversification, I have found that annuities are beneficial.

One other point on picking your Certified Financial Planner. Some of them try to time the financial markets and will buy and sell your assets based on that timing. I have found timing does not work for me over calendar time. Also you may be paying the planner a fee based on each transaction. This reduces your investment amount on a methodology that I have found does not work for me.

Over time you will see your investments grow most of the time. This growth will be maximized through diversification, investment in several different vehicles that vary in asset growth, some in opposite directions, as market conditions change. This variation is one of the reasons to be diversified in your investments. The decline in one area is offset by the increase in another area. The net effect is generally an overall increase in your total portfolio. There may be a time when your overall invested assets decline. Do not panic over this condition. When you are in one of these declines, and they will occur, just look up the growth of the American economy over the last sixty years. I am sure your reaction will be the same as mine which was to only regret I was not able to begin to invest sooner with more assets put into stocks, bonds and the like.

Betting on the American economy over time is, I believe, the best bet in the world.

Another help in escaping your own depression during investment downturns is to have a good Certified Financial Planner, one you have gotten to know, one who has done a good job in recommending investment vehicles and changes in the past. Your CFP needs to become like your doctor. You depend on your doctor to make decisions for you that will prevent serious health problems and let your life extend as far as possible. You depend on your CFP to prevent your financial health from failing and will let your financial life extend to the end of your life.

I went through one of those down turns in the financial markets where my overall invested assets decreased. This was at the time I was paying, even with partial long term care insurance coverage, a substantial amount of money for my wife to be in the assisted living facility. Believe me there were times I became concerned but having a good CFP available to talk to and to reassure me that I would be fine was a tremendous help. I did reduce some of my spending and I delayed purchasing some items during this time but I still enjoyed life and used the assets I did spend in a manner that satisfied all my needs and many of my wants. Today my investments have grown well beyond the decreased amounts.

I have mentioned previously the real necessity for long term care insurance. I believe there really is no other need greater for those who will need long term care. Since we can never know before-hand whether we or a dependent loved one will need such care we all need to acquire long term care insurance. I surely had no idea I would ever need long term care insurance but am I ever glad I had at least partial coverage when my wife was diagnosed with Alzheimer's. After her diagnosis I would not have been able to obtain any long term care insurance coverage.

Many employers offer long term care insurance as group coverage. My employer did but I never really seriously considered getting it as I was very healthy and so, I thought, was my wife. Deciding to not take my employer supplied long term care insurance was a mistake because it would have been cheaper at the group rate and my younger age. When I retired I could have kept the insurance as a retiree. If your employer offers long term care insurance I would highly recommend you seriously examine taking it regardless of your age.

If you do not have and cannot get long term care insurance through your employer than see your CFP or obtain one to get long term care insurance. Many life insurance agents will also be able to offer you long term care policies.

If you or your spouse are fifty years old or older I suggest you need to strongly consider purchasing long term care insurance. My wife was just fifty years old when she began to show the symptoms of Alzheimer's. There are other debilitating diseases which can begin by the age of fifty or younger. Having long term care coverage when any disease of that nature begins will be a real "worry reducer" and asset protector. Also, as with life insurance policies, the younger you are when you purchase the long term care insurance the lower the premiums. At age fifty many have the assets to purchase long term care insurance and pay the premiums, either annually or monthly if the annual cost is larger than you can afford to pay in one payment. For many people age fifty is at the time when your need for significant life insurance has passed so the overall amount of life insurance could be reduced to lower the premiums to help cover the cost of long term care insurance.

The long term care coverage you purchase or currently own needs to cover not only any initial in home care but needs to have an escalator clause to help cover the annual rise in costs of in-facility care.

Long term care insurance costs are continually increasing but will not approach the cost of spending three, four, five or more years in a care facility where costs are also increasing. For example, if a long term care policy costs two thousand dollars per year for each spouse that is forty thousand dollars for a period of twenty years for each of you or a total of eighty thousand dollars for both. If either of you then need in-facility care at eighty thousand dollars per year, and that is a good "ball park" estimate for the present time, then your first year expense equals the cost of the long term care insurance for the both of you over those preceding twenty years. Not a bad investment when you consider in-facility stays usually go well beyond one year. I recently read in Newsweek magazine that the cost of being in a nursing home by the year two thousand twenty five will approximate two hundred and fifty thousand dollars per year. Due to the increase in population and the increase in the age of our population the article called the coming situation the potentially greatest crisis we will face going into the second quarter of this century. To further illustrate the rising costs of long term care, one nursing home I had initially considered for my wife was one hundred and fifty dollars per day at that time. Two years later when I was considering moving my wife to another facility the cost at that same nursing home I had initially considered had increased to two hundred and seventy five dollars per day.

I have read there are some financial quarters that say if you have more than a million dollars in assets you do not need long term care insurance. I believe that, as in my case, the unknown of the future regarding long term illness, the increasing cost of nursing homes and the length of time the illness may last that long term care insurance is a good "investment" regardless of your wealth. The only exception is for those who will be Medicaid qualified from the start of care or soon after.

I did not have enough long term care coverage for my wife. With coverage for in-home care and an escalator clause which automatically increases the amount of in-facility coverage on an annual basis I would have had much more of my assets left in investments even with the increased premiums to cover those added benefits. I have added both in-home care and the escalator clause to my long term care insurance.

There is an important financial item you need to consider that most Certified Financial Planners do not handle. That is determining your tax obligation. CFPs do help you with investing to reduce your taxes. A good accountant (CPA) who keeps up with the tax laws can be very beneficial in determining your taxes each year depending on your income, your expenses and the extent of your assets.

The reason to consider a CPA is that all costs associated with illness and long term care, both in-home and in an outside facility, are today tax deductible. Those deductions are established by Congress and can change at any time. A good CPA will keep up with those changes and be able to get you the most tax reduction based on your particular situation. My taxes were reduced considerably by being able to deduct my out-of-pocket expenses for the care facility and the associated costs of things like diapers, wipes and latex gloves. The deduction also included the cost of long term care insurance.

I have said nothing up to now about your retirement and social security. Whatever your current thinking about the availability of social security when you retire that is not the income goal you want to set when planning for your financial future. Today's social security top pay-out is far from what is required to meet the needs of the current recipients. We read almost daily about the plights bestowed on "fixed income" people when for example taxes increase, fuel costs increase, food costs increase. Your financial security needs to be determined by your management of your finances to meet those needs aided by the counseling of a good CFP. This is true regardless of your current age. Social security then will become an income for which you have much less dependency whatever the pay-out is in future years.

Chapter 6
Staying Mentally and Physically Fit

When I met my wife while I was in college I was physically working out four and five days a week. Through most of our married life I continued to stay physically fit. Through association with positive people and the experiences with my son I also gained more mental strength. Both my physical and mental strength were very helpful assets much later in my life when my wife was diagnosed with Alzheimer's. Physically I, at times, had to carry her from room to room and I had to rearrange furniture to meet her changing needs. Mentally I could have been blown away at the thought of losing my wife much earlier than either of us ever imagined. Both, mental and physical fitness, are required to allow any caregiver to a disabled loved one the ability to provide the best possible care while at the same time keeping themselves healthy.

Much of staying mentally fit has already been covered in previous chapters particularly chapter three on positive thinking. Also, the points about keeping busy doing things you enjoy and being with people you enjoy will be a tremendous help to your mental well being especially in the face of caring for a loved one who has Alzheimer's or any other disease requiring your care.

Many risk factors appear to be associated with lifestyle. The big four lifestyle factors are eat right, exercise, watch your weight and don't smoke. Each factor has an effect on your cardiovascular system which in turn has an effect on your brain health. I read recently about a study by Kaiser Permanente discussed by the editors of AARP magazine that adults in their forties with one or more cardiovascular risk factors were more likely than their peers to develop dementia in their sixties and seventies.

Mental exercise of mind-challenging activities has been shown to lower the risk of dementia. Activities like reading, gardening, playing cards, going to museums, working puzzles, keeping socially active are all boosts to the brain and have some effect on reducing the likelihood to develop Alzheimer's.

What about your physical fitness? Your physical fitness significantly affects your mental fitness. The opposite is also true.

Are you overweight? Do you eat many of the wrong things? Do you not eat enough or too much? Do you exercise little to none? Are you unable to produce all the physical strength you need to accomplish required tasks? Do you get out of breath when climbing a short flight of stairs? Are you always tired? Do you feel you have no energy?

You need to ask yourself these questions. Do that now and be honest with your answers. If you answered "yes" to one or more than I suggest you may need to pay more attention to your physical well being.

Are you presently caring for someone with a disease like Alzheimer's that is requiring much of your energy and time? If so, then you are already experiencing one of the needs for maintaining good physical conditioning. If you are not in good physical condition than you are probably experiencing a level of weariness and maybe even frustration at not being able to meet the physical challenges required in giving the needed care. These can occur for example as you need to lift your loved one, turn them over or just produce the number of steps you will need to take each day in their care. Most people can correct their physical deficiencies.

Those not experiencing a current burden of care taker but who answered "yes" to the questions still need to correct your physical deficiencies for whatever your life's events are at this time and in preparation for upcoming future events that may become adversity in your life. General health improvement should be your goal. As an added incentive, if you need one, to get and stay physically fit is the real deterrent in helping deny or at least delay the onset of many diseases. I have read diseases that can affect the heart, lungs, brain, muscles, bones and digestive tract can be delayed and often avoided in many people by staying physically fit.

.

Of the nine common diseases of Alzheimer's, breast cancer, colorectal cancer, diabetes, heart disease, high cholesterol, hypertension, prostate cancer and stroke, exercise and or diet is mentioned in what you can do to help in the prevention of every one of the nine diseases in many medical journals and current day magazines. Then we need to do two things. One is to learn what a healthy diet is for you and the other is to be on an exercise program. Both of these actions you need to take can be partially addressed by some of what has already been covered in this book and that is to add wholesome activities to your daily regimen to replace inertia. My definition of inertia is the over use of a rocking chair!

I'll address diet first. We have all heard of the many diets reported in several forms of the media that offer us ways to lose weight through changing what and how much we eat. There are several organizations in place that offer us, usually for a fee, ways to reduce our weight by changing what and how much we eat. There are many reports of the success and failure of the diets and these organizations. We have seen that some of the diets actually propose opposite means to weight reduction. Opposing views like eating lo-carbohydrate (lo-carbs) and high protein foods or vice versa. We have all heard the many reports from individuals and the experts that said getting started on a diet is not the problem. The problem is sticking to the diet once started. I believe there are even more people who have never started any diet though one is required to reduce an over weight condition.

I started to gain weight when I was early middle age. I got material on various diet plans available at that time, picked one and tried it. I saw I was losing weight but I was not happy with the methods prescribed in the plan. It seemed to require more than I considered necessary for weight loss. Even so, I was losing weight so I stuck with the plan until I reached my target weight. Then I stopped the diet.

Sometime later I had again gained weight so this time I picked a different plan, one I thought I would better enjoy indulging in. Well, again, I lost weight but was not happy with what I was doing so I stopped the plan until I again had gained the weight back. I was treating my body like a rubber band, stretch it out then let it collapse. I decided I would now lose weight and keep it off permanently. I decided I would keep it off permanently because what I had been doing did not seem too smart for my overall well-being and the number of different sized clothes now filling up my closet was an embarrassment. That also took away an area of gift selection for me because no one had any idea what size of anything to buy me for my birthday or Christmas so my tie collection grew significantly!

To me how I got to my weight and then gained is the same as how most people get to their current weight. How most of you and I got to our weight is a matter of arithmetic, calories in, eaten, versus calories out, burned. No one will deny that our weight is determined by the calories we eat. Most foods we eat have them. If we ingest more calories each day than we remove from our bodies then we gain weight. The opposite follows that if we remove more calories from our bodies each day than we take in then we lose weight. If you are close to your ideal weight at this time then you are taking in about the correct number of calories as you are burning for your size and that is the goal we all must attain to remove being over weight from our list of worries or what should be a worry if you are over weight. Remember the discussion on worry. It does no good, so put together a plan to eliminate the worry and begin to execute the plan now. Focusing on the solution and implementing a plan to obtain the solution will eliminate the worry.

If you are over weight you fall into one of several scenarios. You eat too much and exercise too little or none; you exercise but not enough to balance the calories you take in by over eating; you eat too little but exercise none so you may have become sedentary and the old rocker has you captured. There are other scenarios that do not cause being over weight but are a problem and that is you exercise a lot but eat too little or you do not exercise much but you eat almost nothing. These scenarios may mean you are bulimic and need medical attention. If you fall into these latter categories and are not bulimic then you need a plan to balance your calories in and calories out to achieve and maintain your proper weight. For some, weight gain needs to be the goal, not weight loss.

So what should a typical diet plan to reduce weight look like?

To balance calories first you may need to know how many calories you are ingesting. There are many places to get a chart of the number of calories in a given amount of the variety of foods we eat. You can get the chart from the library, the internet or by just asking your doctor. Actually, for some, probably for most, you will not need this chart because you know you over eat and must reduce calories. You can just eliminate some foods or food quantities without actually counting the calories. For example, if you are overweight and if you eat a large bowl of ice cream almost every night, stop it; if you drink several beers a day, stop it; if you snack between meals, stop it; if you eat a desert after dinner, stop it; if you put heaps of high calorie foods on your plate at one or more of the three meals each day, stop it and take smaller portions. Each of the "stop it's" are really changing a habit you have developed that for most of us is not too difficult to stop once we make the decision to start. Then measure the progress to the goal of losing so many pounds in some amount of time so long as the amount of time is reasonable and not too long or too short. For most people, if you set the goal to lose two pounds a week, that is noticeable after a couple of weeks. That is the goal I was given to achieve during my diets. I always met that goal and exceeded it on many weeks. If you are not achieving the goal then just add some more of the "stop-its" of the type mentioned until you are meeting the goal. You now have a weight reduction plan that is simple and very easy to implement and will be very effective. This is the type of plan I adopted to stop mistreating my body. I ate foods I enjoy at each meal and stopped eating and drinking things that had become pure habit otherwise. I did not bother to count calories and I was doing nothing to dislike. My weight came down and stayed down. Today I eat few things with sugar and trim the fat off of the meats I eat. With that and the changes I made to old eating habits I am able to comfortably maintain a proper weight level with no strict regimen that is not enjoyable. Oh sure, there are times I gorge on delicious meals but after most of those meals I am so uncomfortable that my vow to never gorge like that again lasts for several months before I again make myself uncomfortable by over-eating and repeat the vow.

If you want to actually do the math of calories in versus out, and that can be a good thing in seeing what foods have the highest calories and need to be reduced or eliminated, then get the calorie chart and use it to plan your meals to provide a reduction in calories for weigh loss or an increase in calories for weight gain. When your goal is an increase in calories to gain weight you will need to plan meals with higher calories until you reach your target weight. Weight gain can also be achieved by reversing the "stop its" to your daily eating except maybe the beer "stop it" although my wife needed to gain weigh early in our marriage and her doctor at that time suggested she drink one beer a night. Since drinking beer to her was like taking a bad tasting medicine she did not follow the doctor's advice but even today we hear at times that a couple of beers a day can be good for you.

How many calories need to be reduced when your goal is to lose weight? From the chart, first determine the number of calories you are ingesting each meal each day including any calories you take in between meals. Write down the number of calories and keep the record on a daily basis. Most charts also give you the number of calories needed to sustain any given weight so anything less than that will start weight loss. Many charts also give you the preferred weight per height for males and females and the amount of calorie reduction needed to lose one pound. You can then set your plan to lose so many pounds in so much time. Again two pounds a week seems to be a reasonable target for most people.

We know eating a balanced diet is a must for giving our bodies the right amount of daily nutrition. Vitamin and mineral intake is also a consideration in your diet planning. No matter what you eat most nutritionists agree that vitamin supplements are a good thing. That's not to say supplements should replace a well balanced diet of the right foods but for many of us we can assure a sufficient intake of vitamins and minerals by adding supplements. For men, we are told that added selenium and vitamin E are good for the prostate. For ladies, calcium supplements help with prevention of later age osteoporosis. Calcium has also been shown to be good for the colon in both men and ladies. The vitamin B complexes help maintain good characteristics in the blood. Also, vitamin B complexes and vitamin E are more and more being touted for their help in preventing or delaying the onset of Alzheimer's.

For most people a good multivitamin may be all you need. Then again, there may be some additional vitamins you need with the multivitamin. My suggestion is to see your doctor about any vitamins you may need. To my daily intake of a multivitamin my doctor added vitamin E and selenium for the prostate and calcium and fiber for the colon. I added vitamin C to help with preventing infections and have found the few colds I get seem to be less severe since I started taking vitamin C. There are many other vitamins that have been shown to be good in reducing heart disease and strokes like the anti-oxidant vitamins A and E along with others. Don't forget the added minerals you may also need so do see your doctor for the correct type and amount of supplements you may need.

A word of caution here. Be very careful of some of the herb type supplements you can get at nutrition supplement stores. There have been many reports that some of those supplements are harmful and even deadly to some people so be sure to consult with your physician before taking any of the herb type supplements.

All weight loss does not have to come from changing eating habits. Equally important with reducing food intake is exercise. An exercise program with a healthy diet means the calories reduced are a combination of the fewer calories eaten plus the loss of calories burned during exercise. In addition, exercise provides a lot more benefits to our health then burning calories.

If you currently exercise a minimum of thirty minutes four days a week and have followed your routine for at least six months then you have probably developed the habit needed to maintain your program and have more than likely already seen the tremendous positive effects on your mental and physical health.

If you do not currently exercise than I suggest you need to start on an exercise program whether or not you need to reduce the number of calories that live in your body for the many other benefits of exercise. Benefits like improved cardiovascular health, better muscle tone and strength, better bones, lower blood pressure, aid in stress management, ability to endure the physical requirements of gardening, moving furniture around the room or just plain going upstairs without feeling like you just climbed Mt. Everest.

Some of those benefits are potentially for others than you. Suppose you are obese, sedentary or any of the other body destroying characteristics some people have and you are the main caregiver to an Alzheimer's or other diseased dependent loved one and you have a heart attack or stroke. Now what? You are in the hospital, if you survived, and potentially on a long path to recovery that will prohibit you from caring for your loved one. What will they do? Will some other family member be able to step forward and pick up the task? Even if one or more family members can, you have now "injured" other family members by not taking care of yourself to help prevent the heart attack and now some family member and others have you and the Alzheimer's patient to care for. This is not a good situation and one that potentially could have been prevented if you had taken care of yourself. I can not imagine how my wife would have been taken care of if prior to her entering a care facility I would have become incapacitated with some health problem of my own. It surely would have been a very difficult, maybe even unmanageable, burden for my children. It would also have required many more of my financial assets for in-home care because my children could not have met all of their responsibilities and cared for their mother twenty four/seven.

Most of us have heard that we need to get a doctor's okay before starting any exercise regimen. That is certainly true but if you have to see a doctor specifically for that then you potentially have another problem because you may not have seen a doctor for a long time. If that is the case then make the doctor's appointment now for the okay to exercise but be sure to get a complete physical examination to rule out any disease that may be starting in your body. This is especially true if you are over forty years old and have not had a physical examination to rule out the beginning of some major body break down.

Now you have the okay to begin an exercise program. Where do you start?

There are two kinds of exercise, aerobic and isometric. Aerobic exercise typically moves the muscles in a manner that gets and keeps them agile and toned while increasing the heart rate to a safe level. That safe level is determined by age and can be gotten from a library, on the internet or from your doctor. Aerobic exercise also improves your endurance to last longer in physically challenging endeavors like lifting and supporting a physically disabled loved one.

There are many types of aerobic exercise, some provided by clubs with instructors who control the workout. Jazzercise is one of these clubs. There is a cost for joining these clubs but they are worthwhile organizations to join because they designate the equipment you will need and usually an experienced person will lead each class. Since the sessions are usually group sessions take a friend with you when you get started. That may help you continue the program. There are many other organizations like privately owned gyms, the YMCA and YWCA that have locations with all the equipment you will need and an advisor to help you develop a program. All of these have a cost but a worthwhile cost especially if you have not exercised in the past and therefore do not have the equipment or the know how to develop your own program.

For some people there will not be the time to be away from home for the time needed to adequately perform an exercise program. That can be definitely true for those caring for a helpless loved one at home. To get started at home you will need to purchase your own equipment. To learn what program you will need you can call the local Y's or talk to a fitness instructor. I am sure most will be happy to give you information over the phone if they know your burdened circumstances. Maybe you can even get away for one session a week. That will give you the education you need and provide some respite for you away from home.

Even if you are not caring for a loved one many people will find the convenience of working out at home provides the incentive to continue the program. I used to get my workouts each morning at home before going to work. I continued those morning workouts after I retired and after my wife was diagnosed with Alzheimer's. I also use some of that time, for example when I was on the exercise bicycle, to read some positive material thereby getting both a physical and mental workout at the same time. Of course, there are others who prefer to get away from home and enjoy the camaraderie of others during workouts.

What aerobic workout equipment will you need when starting to workout at home? Not much! Exercises like those performed at Jazzercise only require a mat to lie on. There is other equipment you can get to diversify the Jazzercise type workout but those items can be added after you get started. Some of the other aerobic types of equipment include stationary bicycles, tread mills, rowing machines, cross country ski machines, steppers and a variety of others that are being developed and advertised on Television (TV) every day. The price of each type of aerobic equipment varies widely from under one hundred dollars to well over one thousand dollars. The equipment I use cost me around one hundred dollars to four hundred dollars for each piece. I have used it for well over twenty years and only had my first stationary bicycle break down. All the rest, a rower, a cross-country ski machine, a stepper and a tread mill have lasted for many miles and are still working well today. Remember, aerobic exercise is to increase your heart rate and to keep your muscles "in use" and agile. Any one of the named pieces of equipment will do that. Each does not take up a lot of room so you can put it into a small apartment. Initially a single piece of equipment is the way to begin or continue your exercise program at home even if you have been going to a gym and now find caring for a loved one at home has become a requirement.

There are some advantages I have found to having multiple and different pieces of aerobic exercise equipment. One is the variety of the workout which may help with the monotony some feel during workouts. With multiple pieces of equipment I will spend ten minutes on each of three different pieces which gives the minimum of thirty minutes and helps to break up the time by using different equipment. Multiple pieces of equipment will also usually cause different muscles to be used enhancing your workout.

Another way to stop the monotony of a workout at home is to have the equipment in front of the TV. Actually there are some TV programs that provide thirty minute aerobic type workouts with an instructor leading a class. I find these to be particularly good in the extent of the workout and though not physically in the presence of others you are still working out with others. As these programs do for me, they can provide a kind of competition for you to see if you can keep up with the program's participants. This is also a way for someone starting an aerobic exercise program to get educated on the needs by learning those needs from the instructor on the program. Several TV channels offer the workouts including some of the cable sports channels. Most channels offer these workouts in the morning. Check your local TV listing for time and channel. If you have a recorder connected to your TV you can tape some of the workouts and use them for your continuing workout any time during the day.

    The savings you will realize by getting to and keeping good health probably makes the investment in a piece of aerobic equipment the best investment you will ever make if you use the equipment for at least thirty minutes four days a week. I know you have heard thirty minutes for three days a week is all it takes but I have found that is the very bare minimum to achieve a level of fitness. Actually, to attain near top physical fitness and maintain it I believe most people who work out find the need to work out forty five minutes to an hour five days a week.

    To start your program, use the minimum of thirty minutes for three days a week. That will be better than doing no exercise at all. As you realize the benefits of being fit you will probably decide to add more time. I added a lot more time to my original schedule but every minute proved very beneficial. At the age of a beginning senior citizen I could still run the one hundred yard dash in ten seconds. When even older I went in for a heart stress test and was told that the results of the test I took, the most difficult one, were equivalent to an Olympic sprinter. All of this and always feeling good was all the motivation I needed to continue the program without hesitation. In fact, I got to the point where if I missed a workout for some reason I felt like I had done something wrong. You too can reach this level of dedication if you get started and pay attention to the results and how much better you look and feel then when you were not exercising.

As a part of your workouts you will need to also do some isometric exercises. These are strength building or strength maintenance exercises where you are developing muscle or maintaining some level of muscle development. This type of exercise involves using some form of weight training equipment. As with aerobics, there are places like the private gyms and the Y's that have the equipment and someone there who can help you with developing a weight-training program. That is important so you will be exercising all the muscles in the correct manner. I began my isometric training as a part of my high school football program. I continued these workouts when I went to college so I had a few years to learn what the various exercises were and what muscles they were targeting. There are also gym programs you attended in school which may have given you some education in isometric exercises. If you have none of this and are not able to get away from home for a few sessions with an instructor then, as with aerobics, call a facility like the private gyms or the Y's to get someone knowledgeable to put together a program for you.

Also, as with aerobics, there is a minimum you need at home in the way of equipment so you can do your work outs at home if you desire or if you are not able to get away from home in the first place. The only equipment you typically need for a minimum strength work out is a set, two, of dumbbells and enough disks initially to bring each dumbbell to ten pounds in increments of a pound for most people. You will find that eventually, for many not very long, you will need to increase the number and weight of the disks on your dumbbells. You may find you want to increase your isometric exercising and add barbells or some sort of universal gym but you will need the space and the funds because these items are not inexpensive.

The isometric exercises needed will work, build, the arms to include biceps, triceps and forearms; the chest, pectorals; the shoulders, the deltoids; the neck; the back including the side muscles or lats; the legs though probably not as necessary as the rest because, assuming you do aerobic exercises, most aerobic exercise will primarily use your legs. Plan on thirty minutes three days a week for the isometric exercises. Isometric exercises tear the small tissues of the muscle and that tear needs a day to heal before tearing the muscle again. This tearing is the primary reason we get sore after straining dormant muscles. For most people, once you have been consistent with your isometric workouts for just a short time the muscle becomes conditioned enough for the soreness to go away.

If you have not been doing isometric exercises start with a minimum of weight on the dumb bells, say 1 pound or less on each one. Each exercise will consist of some number of repetitions, reps, in so many sets. The number of sets is usually three and the initial number of reps is a low number to just cause some initial strain, "burn", on the last rep or two. As your muscles get in better condition increase the number of reps to continually get some burn from the last two reps. Once you have gotten to twenty reps then increase the weight. After about six months of isometric exercising you should be able to increase the weight and reduce the number of reps to eight per set for each exercise providing you are still getting burn on the last rep.

Once you develop the muscles to the size you are comfortable with decrease the weight and increase the reps so you are now maintaining the muscle but not building it larger. Of course if initially you only want to maintain any given muscle size then start in the beginning and continue with lighter weigh and more reps per set.

The first few years I had done isometric exercises I was in the muscle building category. I continued to add weight to my exercise routines and to build muscle. Once I even entered the Mister Virginia contest though I was more interested in getting that time away from college to see my future wife than I was in pumping my muscles in front of a crowd of people. In fact, that experience was not something I ever wanted to repeat and I didn't. Soon after this I was playing baseball and found I could not any longer swing the bat level. I could still hit the ball but I only knocked it a country mile into the air giving all three out-fielders enough time to set up camp under the ball before catching it for an out. That caused me to realize I had overdone the muscle building. I then reduced the weigh on all of my isometric exercises and increased the number of reps. That eventually got me back to the level of coordination I had lost.

As you get older and enter the senior citizen category you will need to reduce any heavy weight to the maintenance only level. I learned this from my physician after I entered the golden, and they are, years. At one of my annual physicals my physician was reviewing my history to update it and asked about my weight training. I said, "Yes, I still do that three times a week along with the five days a week of aerobics." He then asked about the weight I was using. Now I am sure he must have noted that I was again increasing in size, as I did in college, to a rather large muscular body. I replied with the amount of weight I was using. He looked at me, I wasn't sure if it was amazement or at my stupidity. I soon found it was the latter, as he asked, "What are you trying to prove?" Without allowing me the chance to answer he continued, "Do you know you could pop a vessel, break a bone or even worse at your age?" Now you have to know I had a lot of respect for this physician so I did not become insulted. Rather I told him I would reduce the weight because I was doing the exercises to live longer, not to shorten my life. I tell you this story to pass on my experience and to give you the same warning particularly if you are now a senior citizen or will soon be a senior citizen and are using or plan to use too heavy a weight in your isometric routines.

You will be amazed at how good you feel once you get into consistent workouts with both aerobic and isometric exercising and continue for just a couple of months. You will also be amazed at how your vital signs including heart rate, blood pressure and lung capacity have improved after just six months. You can verify this by getting a follow up check of these vital signs from your physician. This coupled with the weight loss included from your diet should really be enough to convince you to stay with proper eating and exercise for the rest of your life.

If that isn't enough then set your goals and reward yourself each time you reach a planned plateau with dates toward reaching your goals. For the guys the reward can be a new fishing rod or a new golf club or whatever your entertainment likes happen to be. For the ladies a new piece of jewelry or a new dress or whatever your likes are for your personal enjoyment. Well sure, some ladies may want to get a new fishing rod or a new golf club. Do any of you guys want a new dress for your lady as your reward? Think about it. That could be a rewarding thing for you to do for you!

The need for proper diet and exercise is required for everyone, men and women. For both, diet and exercise, men and women need to get their physicians approval of any program they begin. The exercises in the isometric weight training programs need to be determined by a professional before beginning to perform them unless you have had previous training.

Of added importance for the care giver to a loved one, with the proper diet and exercise routines you will have found a way to look forward to something on a several times a week basis and will have developed a very beneficial activity at home to help occupy some time.

Conclusion

I have written this book with the hope it will have some positive effect on the reader, particularly the reader who is now caring for or who in the future may have to care for a loved one with Alzheimer's or some other disease that causes total or almost total reliance on someone else for survival.

The subject matter in the book is a documentation of my experiences and knowledge gained, my installed learning through repetition, in the various subjects. My knowledge in these subjects includes information from professionals and information provided in the many books I have read, many of which are referenced in the appendix. Of course, my actual hands on experiences with the subject matter in each chapter have been the best teacher for the advice I offer in the book.

I have experienced and continue to experience the benefits of what I have said about positive thinking, financial planning and staying fit. My assets, started when my wife and I were first married, are still growing and providing me with my life-style needs and wants. I have updated information available to me on an on going basis of all legal and important information my agent or I may need on a moment's notice. I experienced the topics on care for a loved one and all the subject matter on that topic up until my wife and her father passed away. God is still working in my life providing me with the desire each morning to enjoy each day learning and participating with my surviving family and friends in many activities including the once a week music sessions. My buddy dog "Bear" has passed away, a very sad time for me, but I now have a Lab puppy named "Bear's Shadow." Shadow is right now lying at my feet and already providing me with the same enjoyment I received from Bear though Bear will never be forgotten.

It is my hope you have at least been energized to the point of thinking about starting some or all of the topics I have covered that are not now a part of your life. If you are not sure of some of what I have said and want to talk to a professional on the subject then please do so but do so now while the spark of the desire is still present. Those early sparks are most often extinguished with the sprinkle of a very short time lapse. Consult any current professional you may have on any of the subjects, use the phone book to locate contact information, use the internet or ask a friend for recommendations. These are all good places to start to find answers to your questions or to locate a professional to get the answers. Just be sure to get references and credentials before paying any fees for advice or training from professionals you did not previously know.

Make adversity or just the possibility that adversity may enter your life work for you by considering doing the things I mention in this book. This will not eliminate the very heart wrenching pain you will feel during some very adverse situations but it will surely help prevent compounding the adversity with needless other worries. You will be able to soar above adversity.

I have enjoyed speaking with you through this medium and I wish for you a long and healthy life free of severe adversity and a life made even happier through the knowledge you are better prepared for adversity should it occur. Good bye!

Appendix A

This is a recommended list of books to read listed by chapter. They are not in any necessary order to obtain the most from each book. I have read most of the books listed and then some. If you read any of the books listed here and practice what you read I believe you will be well on your way toward being better able to handle most adversity.

*Chapter 1—Alzheimer's the Beginning to the End
1. For readers with Alzheimer's or care takers who have a loved one with Alzheimer's call your local Alzheimer's Association for their recommended book list. They will lend you several of their recommended books.
2. *Tough Times Never Last But Tough People Do* by Robert H. Schuller

*Chapter 2—Spiritual Guidance
1. The Holy Bible
    —Old Testament
    —Old and New Testament
2. *The Purpose Driven Life* by Rick Warren

3. *Be Happy You Are Loved* by Robert H. Schuller
4. *The Greatest Miracle in the World* by Og Mandiino
5. *When Bad Things Happen to Good People* by Harold Kushner

*Chapter 3—The Power of Positive Thinking

You can look up the quotes used in this chapter by referencing the following:
1. brainyquotes.com
2. Laura Moncur's Motivational Quotations
3. Cole's Quotables
4. quotationspage.com
5. WorldofQuotes.com

The following are all texts:
1. *7 Habits of Highly Successful People* by Stephen R. Covey
2. *The Miracle Success System* by Forrest H. Frantz, Sr.
3. *Seeds of Greatness* by Denis Waitley
4. *See You At The Top* by Zig Ziglar
5. *Peace of Mind Through Possibility Thinking* by Robert H. Schuller
6. *The Power of Positive Thinking* by Norman Vincent Peale
7. *The Magic Power of Self-Image Psychology* by Maxwell Maltz
8. *Psychocybernetics* by Maxwell Maltz
9. *Getting the Most Out of Life—An Anthology* from Readers Digest
10. *Think and Grow Rich* by Napoleon Hill
11. *I Can* by Ben Sweetland
12. *I Will* by Ben Sweetland
13. *Grow Rich While You Sleep* by Ben Sweetland

14. *How to Win Friends and Influence People* by Dale Carnegie
15. *Enthusiasm Makes the Difference* by Norman Vincent Peale
16. *You Can If You Think You Can* by Norman Vincent Peale
17. *Successful Living Day by Day* by Nelson Boswell
18. *What You say Is What You Get* by Don Gossett
19. *What to Say When You Talk to Yourself* by Shad Helmstetter, Phd
20. *The Magic of Getting What You Want* by David A. Schwartz
21. *The Magic of Thinking Big* by David A. Schwartz
22. *Life Is Tremendous* by Charlie Jones
23. *How to Stop Worrying and Start Living* by Dale Carnegie
24. *The Magic of Believing* by Claude M. Bristol
25. *Wake Up and Live* by Dorothea Brande
26. *Living Without Losing* by Don Polston
27. *The Magic of Self Direction* by David J. Schwartz, Phd

*Chapter 4—Legal and Administrative Needs

You can find information in this chapter in the library legal section or on the internet. This will provide you with any additional material you need on wills, living wills, HCPOAs, trusts and powers-of-attorney. I have not read any specific texts on what I learned about my legal needs. I have read many articles on the many subjects. I was educated directly by my attorney and by my experience in obtaining and using the documents and information I relate in the book.

*Chapter 5—Building and Maintaining Your Assets
1. *Burning Money* by J. Peter Grace
2. *Personal Money Management* by Thomas E. Bailard, David L. Biehl, Ronald W. Kaiser
3. *The Power of Being Debt Free* by Robert H. Schuleller and Paul David Dunn
4. *The Real Estate Investment Pocket Guide* by Alan J. Parisse, Richard G. Wollack
5. *Money Dynamics* by Anita VanClaspel
6. *How to Be Rich* by J. Paul Getty
7. *The Wall Street Journal Lifetime Guide to Money* edited by C. Frederic Wiegold, personal finance editor
8. *Cut Your Bills In Half* by the editors of Rodale Press

*Chapter 6—Stay Mentally and Physically Fit
1. *You Can Feel Good All the Time* by Robert D. Willix, Jr. MD
2. "Men's Health" or "Woman's Health" magazines. These have a subscription cost but are very good in covering various topics on physical health.

CPSIA information can be obtained at www.ICGtesting.com
Printed in the USA
BVOW011813061011

273021BV00002B/1/P